The
MD Factor
Diet

The MD Factor Diet

A PHYSICIAN'S PROVEN DIET FOR METABOLISM CORRECTION AND HEALTHY WEIGHT LOSS

Caroline J. Cederquist, M.D.

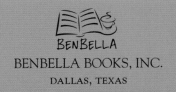

BENBELLA

BENBELLA BOOKS, INC.

DALLAS, TEXAS

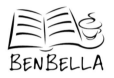

BenBella Books, Inc.
10300 N. Central Expressway
Suite #530
Dallas, TX 75231
www.benbellabooks.com
Send feedback to feedback@benbellabooks.com

Printed in the United States of America
10 9 8 7 6 5 4 3 2 1

Library of Congress Cataloging-in-Publication Data is available upon request.
978-1-941631-28-7

Cover and interior design by Matt Mayerchak
Interior composition by PerfecType, Nashville, TN
Cover and interior photography by Erik Keller Photography
Illustrations on pages 27, 33, 38, 39, 128, 129, 181, and 215 by Jim Atherton
Proofreading by Jessika Rieck and Clarissa Phillips
Printed by Versa Press

Distributed by Perseus Distribution
www.perseusdistribution.com

To place orders through Perseus Distribution:
Tel: (800) 343-4499
Fax: (800) 351-5073
E-mail: orderentry@perseusbooks.com

Significant discounts for bulk sales are available. Please contact Glenn Yeffeth at glenn@benbellabooks.com or (214) 750-3628.

Contents

About the Author

Dr. Caroline J. Cederquist is one of only 850 physicians who have achieved a board certification in bariatric medicine. She has conducted years of clinical research and specializes in nutrition and metabolism. She is a nationally recognized and versatile media personality covering a wide spectrum of health-related news and topics.

After graduating from the University Of Miami School of Medicine, she completed her residency and board certification in family medicine. In 1998, she opened her practice, Cederquist Medical Wellness Center, in Naples, Florida. Based on requests from a rapidly expanding client base, in 2005 she cofounded bistroMD, a national weight loss company that provides physician-designed, chef-prepared weight loss meals that are delivered to your home.

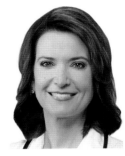

Caroline J. Cederquist, M.D.

Dr. Cederquist provides an opportunity for a wellness transformation to patients who have metabolism dysfunction. She helps patients with complex medical conditions related to weight and nutritional issues. She also identifies and treats food allergies and sensitivities, giving access to her patients to feel well—sometimes for the first time. Her practice strives to give patients the path to a vibrant, healthy lifestyle through nutrition, metabolism correction, weight loss, and weight management.

Through her practice and media outreach, she aims to help men, women, and children through the struggles and confusion of weight management with the identification and treatment of metabolism dysfunction.

Career Highlights Include:

- Author of *Helping Your Overweight Child, A Family Guide*
- Contributor to national television including *Dr. Phil, Ricki Lake,* and *NBC News*
- Regular contributor editor for *Huffington Post* and *è Bella Magazine*
- Recognized as an expert in numerous print and e-publications, including the *New York Times, Wall Street Journal, Time, CNN, Glamour, Shape, Men's Health, Elle, Woman's Day, Family Circle, Parenting Magazine, Men's Fitness,* and *Health Magazine*

- Former Trustee, American Society of Bariatric Physicians
- National Upjohn Achievement Award recipient for Outstanding Academic and Personal Qualities in a Physician
- Keynote Speaker for national and regional wellness seminars including Metabolic Summit
- Officer of Alpha Omega Alpha Medical Society

Dr. Cederquist is also a busy mom of four and devoted to her husband, Ed, fondly referred to as The Foodie and cofounder of bistroMD. The duo combines the science of healthy weight loss with their passion for great tasting, nutritious food to create a compelling difference in people's lives.

Our Charter

Cederquist Medical Wellness Center partners with our patients to create a profound transformation that makes a lifelong difference in their health and well-being.

We are experts in nutrition and metabolism. Firmly grounded in medical science, we are a refreshing opportunity for our patients who have difficulty obtaining an optimally functioning metabolism. We strive to continuously refine and explore the medical and metabolic reasons why achieving and maintaining a healthy weight can be so challenging for our patients who have achieved success and mastery in almost every other aspect of their lives.

We stand for that all people's well-being can be transformed. Many, while hopeful for change, come to us resigned by the difficulties and issues they have known. Some feel their body has changed and a new frustrating metabolism has taken over. Others have had issues for as long as they can remember and find it difficult to visualize a different future. A number of our patients share that they do not know and never have known what it is like to feel well. We acknowledge and appreciate the strength, courage, and integrity necessary to triumph over these health challenges. Our partnership powerfully enables our patients to let go of ineffective nutrition plans and patterns of behavior that no longer work within the context of a healthy future.

Our excitement with our work goes beyond healthy weight management. With thorough investigation and analysis and the collaboration of our patients, our multidisciplinary team creates a carefully devised plan of action to alleviate or significantly improve physical symptoms that dampen vitality, as well as create a new future of health and well-being.

We recruit and develop dynamic, skillful professionals who are committed to the lives we touch and the pursuit of excellence.

It is our fortune to play an integral role in the successes and accomplishments that impact our patient's lives.

Our patients are able to obtain a quality of life that had been lost or was never known and confidently embrace a new vibrant and healthy future.

Acknowledgments

Putting more than twenty years of what you do day to day into a book should be so easy and straightforward. However, it was a great undertaking and I am so grateful to the many people who helped put into words the motivating and refreshing opportunity I am privileged to provide for my patients on a daily basis.

First, I must thank my husband, Ed Cederquist, for always supporting me in my desire to create a medical practice dedicated to nutrition and metabolism unlike any other in existence. This support also created bistroMD, the amazing home meal delivery program that allows the benefits of my knowledge and expertise to touch hundreds of thousands of people outside of my practice. I thank my four beautiful and amazing children, two of whom are now adults. Thank you for trying the meals created for our programs because we always knew a "thumbs up" from you signaled a winning recipe. Thank you for patiently sharing me with my work, research, and writing. I thank my parents, Cathy and Neale Szabo. You always supported me in everything I wanted to pursue, including my plan to become a physician.

Thank you to Adriana Kinn, the brilliant nurse practitioner I have been blessed to work with for the past twelve years. Your attention to detail and greatly skilled, insightful, and motivating coaching has helped thousands of our patients. Thank you to the dynamic and skillful team of dietitians at Cederquist Medical Wellness Center—Joy Post, Nicole Hartwick, Amy Geant, Natasha Genevro, and others over the years. You take the nutrition prescription to correct metabolism dysfunction and turn it into a meal plan that our patients enjoy eating. Thank you for partnering with our patients to create a profound transformation that makes a lifelong difference in their health and well-being. Thank you to my administrative and support team at the medical center—Rebecca and Julie. Thank you for your dedication to the people we serve and your pursuit of excellence. Thank you as well to Donna Alpert, LMHC, who for the past twelve years has shared her wisdom and solutions with those patients who have struggled with patterns of behavior that no longer work in the context of a healthy future.

With regards to the book specifically, a further great thank-you goes to Joy Lynn Post. You and I created the first manuscript that would eventually become *The MD Factor Diet*. Your nutritional knowledge coupled with your gift for making it understandable on paper is such a brilliant combination, and I am so thankful for all you have contributed to the educational modules of the medical center, as well as to this book. I expect further great things as you complete your doctoral degree in nutrition and add more to the field.

Thank you, Rebecca Wells and Wesley Bloemers. Your brilliance in writing and marketing at such a young age is humbling. Thank you for championing this book project and taking it from pages of medical jargon and dietary data to the beautiful and user-friendly book it is today. Thank you, Sonja Pustay, for your contributions to the editing process. Thank you to my business coach Kelly Townsend for your talents in helping us create the charters of the Cederquist Medical Wellness Center and bistroMD and for coaching us to fulfill on those charters.

Thank you to dietitian Sarah Hallenberger and to the chefs of bistroMD for your insights and for sharing some of the fabulous recipes of bistroMD with our readers.

Thank you, Karen Moline, for your upbeat and motivational writing style. You made what I say come alive in the written format. Thank you to Mayerchak & Co. for the skillful book design and production. The artistic design and clean organizational style reflect how doable correcting the **MD Factor** is for people.

Thank you to my great friend Rebecca Zung-Clough for your friendship and the fact that I am always empowered in your presence.

Finally, I thank my patients and the medical community of Collier County. I have been so fortunate over the years to have had thousands of men, women, children, and their physicians entrust me and my team with their care and the creation of their new healthy futures. You are my motivation to always research more and learn more about the mysteries of metabolism and the healing power of clean, great-tasting, nourishing food.

—C.J.C.

The
MD Factor
Diet

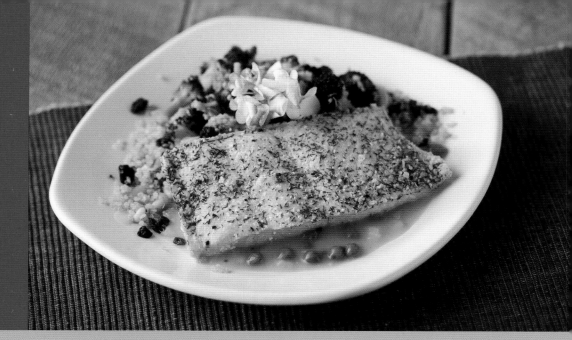

Salmon piccata with couscous and broccoli

PART I

DISCOVER YOUR MD FACTOR

CHAPTER 1

Metabolism Dysfunction: It's Not Your Fault

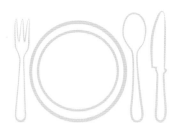

"Why is it so hard for me to lose weight?"

That's the question I hear every day from patients who've come to my weight management medical practice. These are smart people who have usually been eating the same amount of food and who are often following strict diets. Many of them have upped their workouts, too, but the weight still won't come off—or, worse, they are gaining weight for seemingly no reason at all! They are incredibly frustrated because they think the only way to lose weight is to eat less and exercise more—which is what the media (and sometimes their physicians) tell them over and over again.

Other patients have become resigned to being overweight, because losing the extra pounds has become too difficult for them. *"I know what to do,"* they'll tell me, *"and I've done it. But it's not working."* Maybe somehow they're eating more than they realize, or they're getting less exercise than they think. Or maybe it's menopause that's making them fat. In any case, they think there's nothing they can do about it.

And some patients tell me, with a heartbreaking look in their eyes, *"I've had a weight problem all my life, and nothing will ever work for me."*

After twenty years of treating patients who want to lose weight, I know exactly why they're so frustrated and upset. They might have put on fat in their torso, especially their bellies. It might creep up slowly or seemingly appear overnight. But these weight problems aren't just about overeating or underexercising—they're about metabolic changes.

In other words, if you've tried to lose weight and haven't made any real progress, one thing is certain: your metabolism has changed. It's like a switch has been flipped and your old, familiar metabolism has been

replaced with a frustratingly difficult new one, a metabolism that likes storing fat. You have what I call the *MD Factor*.

The **MD Factor** is incredibly common:

✔ When you gain belly weight for any reason, your metabolism changes.

✔ When you have hormonal changes, your metabolism changes.

✔ As you age, your metabolism changes.

You don't have to be overweight to have the **MD Factor**. Even if your weight is perfectly normal, you can still suffer from its effects. This is particularly important for premenopausal women to know, as following the **MD Factor** Action Plan you'll read about in this book can help prevent the typical fifteen-to-thirty-pound weight gain that happens around menopause.

Let me tell you that your symptoms are very real. Craving sugars, feeling foggy, having energy dips throughout the day, and increased hunger are all symptoms of the **MD Factor**. I know how hard it is to lose weight if you are hungry, have intense cravings, and have no energy. After following the **MD Factor** Plan for just one week, these symptoms will be better.

The **MD Factor** is caused by changes in how your body is able to use the nutrients in your food, and even though it's very common, it's not often recognized by those who have it—or by their physicians. Whatever your weight, when your metabolism is no longer acting the way it used to, you can fix it. There is a specific way your body needs to be fed to get the best out of your metabolism, ensuring that you are able to lose weight and keep it off. You'll see how to do just that with the **MD Factor** Action Plan.

Even if you've tried every diet out there and not lost the weight you wanted, the **MD Factor** Action Plan will work for you. You can lose

Even if you've tried every diet out there and not lost the weight you wanted, the **MD Factor** Action Plan will work for you.

What have you got to lose? Nothing but a lot of weight, a lot of health problems, and a lot of frustration!

weight and keep it off. That's because the **MD Factor** Action Plan is not merely a diet—it's a lifestyle change that works. It will empower you to lose weight, as well as prevent future weight gains.

The **MD Factor** Action Plan gives you access to a healthy future. By adjusting your diet and lifestyle, you'll eat better, sleep better, have more energy, be sharper and more focused, and lower your risk for heart disease, some cancers, stroke, and dementia.

What have you got to lose? Nothing but a lot of weight, a myriad of health problems, and a lot of frustration!

How the **MD Factor** Can Impact Your Health

I decided to become a physician because I wanted to help people live the healthiest lives possible. I graduated from medical school in 1991 and completed specialized training in family practice, learning how to care for people from infancy through childhood, adolescence, and adulthood, during pregnancy, through the years of hormone changes such as menopause, and through all aspects of aging.

I realized early on that many of my patients had medical problems and a decreased quality of life due to problems with their weight. I decided I would learn everything I could about nutrition and metabolism to help them live healthier and more vibrant lives. I have years of clinical experience with thousands of patients of all ages—men, women, and children. I've also spent years researching why metabolism can become dysfunctional and why losing weight can become so difficult even for highly motivated people. To better help them, I created the comprehensive Cederquist Medical Wellness Center, where I'm aided by my expert team of dietitians, a nurse practitioner, a behavioral therapist, and exercise specialists.

It is incredibly gratifying to see a patient radiate joy and triumph after dropping several dress sizes or getting a smaller belt. It's wonderful to see these physical signs of a metabolism that is now working again. But because I am a physician first, I know that while helping people look better is great, there is more to my mission in life. I have become an expert in nutrition and metabolism for another reason: correcting the **MD Factor** can have many benefits. It adds years to my patients' lives, helps their medical conditions, and reduces the medications they are required to take.

Here's how an uncontrolled **MD Factor** can negatively impact your health:

✔ **It increases your risk of heart disease.** The **MD Factor** is one of the major reasons cholesterol levels get skewed, with too many triglycerides and too little "good" HDL cholesterol. This abnormal cholesterol profile, or dyslipidemia, is a major contributor to heart disease, which leads to heart attacks. The **MD Factor** also increases inflammation, a newly discovered risk factor for heart attacks.

✔ **It increases your risk of stroke.** A stroke impedes blood flow to your brain. It can cause permanent brain and nerve damage, and even kill you.

✔ **It increases your risk of high blood pressure.** This makes it more likely that you'll develop heart disease or have a stroke later in life.

✔ **It increases your risk for type 2 diabetes.** Type 2 diabetes is almost always caused by lifestyle, particularly by being overweight. Diabetes is an extremely serious illness and is a leading cause of blindness, kidney disease, heart disease, circulatory problems, and general disability. The longer you have it, the more damage it can do to your organs. And the disease is now reaching epidemic levels: as of 2011, 27 percent of adults over sixty-five in America have diabetes, and 35 percent of Americans over twenty have

I've also spent years researching why metabolism can become dysfunctional and why losing weight can become so difficult even for highly motivated people.

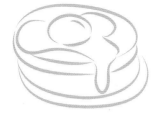

pre-diabetes, which means they've had the **MD Factor** for years and are at grave risk for developing diabetes. And most of them don't know they have it.

The **MD Factor** also greatly increases your risk for many other ailments:

- ✔ **Cancer:** breast cancer, colon cancer, endometrial cancer, esophagus cancer, gallbladder cancer, kidney cancer, leukemia (in adults), liver cancer, lymphoma, pancreatic cancer, prostate cancer

- ✔ **Dementia** and other forms of mental decline

- ✔ **Kidney disease**

- ✔ **Nerve damage**

Take heart, though. You can fight and defeat the **MD Factor** and successfully reverse many of these health risks.

Is This You?

You'll be able to pinpoint your **MD Factor** symptoms in more detail once you take the quiz on page 9, but see if you have any of these:

❑ You crave sugary foods, and once you start eating them, you find it difficult to stop.

❑ You feel weak or light-headed after missing a meal or shortly after having something sweet on an empty stomach. (For example, if you eat a doughnut at 8:00 a.m., you'll feel weak or foggy an hour later.)

❑ You have afternoon energy slumps several hours after lunch.

❑ You have a hard time sleeping soundly through the night. You tend to wake up a few hours after falling asleep, then feel too wide awake to be able to get back to sleep.

❑ You have trouble focusing and maintaining attention.

❑ You have frequent mood swings.

❑ If you are a woman in your midforties or beyond, you may experience hot flashes.

❑ You feel that if you don't have something to eat at the exact moment that hunger pangs strike, you'll be grumpy, edgy, light-headed, or shaky.

❑ You want to eat pasta, rice, or other starchy carbohydrates at meals. You crave potato chips, popcorn, sweets, cookies, candy, or crackers.

❑ You eat cereal with milk and fruit for breakfast, yet find you are starving by 10:00 a.m.—hungrier than if you skipped breakfast altogether.

❑ Your hunger is so intense at 5:00 or 6:00 p.m. that you think, "I'll eat anything that doesn't eat me first!"

❑ You find it extremely difficult to lose weight and very easy to gain weight.

These patients are almost always shocked—and then relieved—that a very real *metabolic* condition has made weight loss so challenging for them.

The **MD Factor** is very frustrating—but you can defeat it. I say that with certainty because I've treated thousands of men, women, and children who've had it, and they've finally won the weight loss battle. I know you can do it, too.

What I want you to do now is take the **MD Factor** Quiz on the next page. I developed it to help you see how the **MD Factor** affects you. Then, in Part II, you'll discover what the **MD Factor** is in more depth. In Part III, you can move right into the **MD Factor** Action Plan. I'll guide you every step of the way. Part IV will give you amazingly delicious recipes, and finally, the appendices have additional information to help you control your **MD Factor**.

So let's get to work!

The **MD Factor** Quiz

Since between 89–94 percent of the patients who come to see me for help with their weight have the **MD Factor**, I developed this quiz to help me pinpoint their symptoms. These patients are almost always shocked—and then relieved—that a very real *metabolic* condition has made weight loss so challenging for them.

As you take the **MD Factor** Quiz, see if any of these symptoms resonate with you. The scoring will help you determine if you have the **MD Factor**. I developed this test in my medical practice and ran clinical studies to test it. My patients' scores on the quiz directly correlated to whether or not they had the **MD Factor** on blood work testing and also how severe their **MD Factor** was. Take the quiz and then check your score in the pages that follow.

The MD Factor Quiz: Part 1

Please circle ONLY ONE of the following answers that most closely describes how you feel every day. Then circle the point value for each answer in the table on the side of the page. Record your points for each question in the table on page 15.

1. **Describe your appetite in the morning.**

   a. I wake up hungry and need breakfast to start my day.

   b. I'm not hungry at first, but in a few hours I need to eat.

   c. I'm mildly hungry and feel better if I have breakfast, but I could go without it if needed.

   d. I have no appetite in the morning. It's really hard for me to be able to eat any breakfast.

2. **How would you describe your energy level at 3:00 p.m.?**

   a. My energy is good.

   b. I'm a little tired, but I can shake it off by getting up and stretching or taking a brief walk away from my desk.

   c. I need a pick-me-up, so I'll look for something with caffeine or a sugary snack.

   d. I'm exhausted. I need a nap, and if I can take one, I'll conk right out.

3. **What's your opinion about sweets such as cookies or starchy foods such as breads or pasta?**

   a. I can take them or leave them. When I have them, fine, but I don't crave them.

   b. I have always liked sugars and starches and still do. No meal is complete without starches as well as dessert.

   c. I like these foods, but I know they're a problem. Every time I eat them, they either increase my appetite or make me hungrier.

   d. I have uncontrollable cravings for sugars and starches even if I've just eaten and am not really hungry. It's almost as if it doesn't matter what the food is or how much I like it or not—I *have* to eat it.

QUESTION 1

Answer	Points
(A)	0
B	1
C	3
D	7

QUESTION 2

Answer	Points
(A)	0
B	1
C	3
D	7

QUESTION 3

Answer	Points
A	0
B	2
C	5
(D)	7

The MD Factor Quiz: Part 2

Please select the answer that best describes how you feel. If you no longer eat or drink the way the question references, then answer how you would have felt in the past when you ate or drank that way.

QUESTION 4

Answer	Points
A	0
B	2
C	7
(D)	7
E	7
F	0

QUESTION 5

Answer	Points
A	0
(B)	3
C	5
D	7
E	7
F	0

4. **How do you feel after eating a typical high-carbohydrate breakfast (cereal, fruit juice, toast, waffles, a bagel, pancakes)?**

   a. I feel good, have lots of energy, and am full.

   b. I feel full but get hungry again a few hours later—usually before my scheduled lunchtime.

   c. I feel crummy. I get tired and don't feel satisfied, so I start looking for something else to eat a few hours later.

   d. This breakfast stimulates my appetite, and I'm ravenous within an hour or two.

   e. This does not apply to me as I never eat this type of breakfast. In the past when I ate this type of breakfast, I had some symptoms of increased appetite.

   f. This does not apply to me as I never eat this type of breakfast. I do not like this type of breakfast, but when I have eaten these foods in the past, I do not recall any symptoms of increased appetite.

5. **How do you feel if you haven't eaten for six or more hours?**

   a. I'm hungry and want to eat, but I can take the time to prepare a healthful meal if it takes less than thirty minutes.

   b. I'm very hungry and can't wait to prepare a meal, so I'll start snacking because I need to eat before my meal is ready.

   c. I feel irritable and cranky or headachy, and I need to get something *fast*.

   d. I feel terrible. I'm weak and shaky and almost feel like I'm going to faint. Basically, I'll eat anything that won't eat me first! And I'll eat it very quickly so I can make that awful feeling go away.

   e. This does not apply to me as I never go this long without eating. In the past, when I went this long without eating, I would get some of the symptoms listed above.

   f. This does not apply to me as I never go this long without eating. In the past, when I went this long without eating, I do not recall having symptoms of hunger, headaches, irritability, or feeling weak.

6. **How do you feel when eating something sweet, such as cookies, or something starchy, such as potatoes or pasta?**

   a. I feel fine. I enjoy these foods and feel satisfied with a normal-size serving.

   b. Sometimes eating these types of food seem to make me hungrier, and I want another portion.

   c. Usually when I eat these types of food, I end up eating slightly more than I wanted, but I don't have to finish every last chip in the bag or the entire box of cookies.

   d. If I eat these foods, I know I won't be able to stop. They make me feel out of control, and I'll eat the whole bag or box no matter how big it is. Even when I'm uncomfortably full, it's really hard to stop eating.

   e. This does not apply to me as I don't eat sweet or starchy food. In the past when I ate these foods, I would have symptoms of increased hunger or loss of control.

   f. This does not apply to me as I don't eat sweet or starchy food. They don't cause any symptoms that I am aware of; I just don't like these foods.

7. **If you eat a meal that contains mostly carbohydrates, such as pasta and garlic bread, how do you feel RIGHT afterward?**

   a. I feel full but otherwise fine.

   b. I feel a little tired shortly after eating.

   c. I feel very physically tired.

   d. I feel like I'm in a mental fog—what I would describe as a food coma—and I want to go to sleep.

   e. This does not apply to me as I don't eat high carbohydrate meals like this. In the past, when I ate meals like this, I felt more physically or mentally tired.

   f. This does not apply to me as I don't eat high carbohydrate meals like this. When I have eaten a meal like this in the past, it did not cause any symptoms that I recall. I just do not like this type of meal.

QUESTION 6

Answer	Points
(A)	0
B	2
C	5
D	7
E	7
F	0

QUESTION 7

Answer	Points
A	0
B	2
C	5
D	7
E	7
(F)	0

QUESTION 8

Answer	Points
Ⓐ	0
B	2
C	7
D	5
E	7
F	7
G	0

8. **How do you feel several hours after that same carbohydrate-rich evening meal, adding a glass of wine to it?**

   a. I feel fine, no different from any other meal.

   b. I feel fine and sleep well. I could be a bit hungrier than usual in the morning.

   c. My sleep is disturbed. I'll wake up in the middle of the night, maybe around 2:00 or 3:00 a.m., and feel wide awake.

   d. I wake up multiple times during the night. I could be a bit hungrier than usual in the morning.

   e. A few hours later I feel warm and sweaty, almost like I'm having a hot flash.

   f. I no longer drink alcohol, but when I did in the past, if combined with a carbohydrate-rich meal, I recall having disturbed sleep or hot flashes.

   g. This does not apply to me as I do not drink alcohol or have carbohydrate-rich meals. If I did have alcohol in the past with a similar meal, I do not recall any effect on my sleep or hot flashes.

The MD Factor Quiz: Part 3

Please circle ONLY ONE of the choices for each question.

9. **If you've tried to lose weight recently, were you successful?**

   a. Yes. I was able to lose weight fairly easily by increasing my exercise and cutting back on portion size, sweets, and alcohol.

   b. Yes, but I can lose weight only if I follow a fairly rigid, structured diet and increase my exercise level. Merely cutting back on food and increasing exercise doesn't work.

   c. Not really. I can lose very slowly if I never cheat on a rigid, low-calorie diet and add a lot more daily exercise to my routine. I should show a lot more results for my efforts. And as soon as I go off the diet, I put on a few pounds really quickly.

   d. No. I'm following such a strict diet that's there's no way I can cut back further, plus I'm exercising more than I ever used to, but I've lost almost no weight. Or, worse, I even gained a few pounds.

   e. This does not apply to me as I have not tried to lose weight recently.

10. **How would you rate your current body weight?**

    a. Very good. I'm at a healthy weight.

    b. I am not necessarily overweight, but I have noticed more weight in my abdominal area, which I did not have before.

    c. I'm slightly overweight.

    d. I am pretty overweight, at least thirty pounds or more over where I should be.

11. **How would you describe how your body stores fat?**

    a. My weight is normal and my body fat is evenly distributed.

    b. I carry any excess weight in my lower body, such as around my hips or thighs.

    c. I am carrying excess body fat and it seems to be evenly distributed, with some in my abdomen and or torso and some in my arms and lower body.

    d. My weight gain is predominantly in my abdomen or my torso, concentrated in my belly, breasts, or back.

QUESTION 9

Answer	Points
A	0
B	5
C	7
(D)	7
E	0

QUESTION 10

Answer	Points
A	0
B	7
(C)	5
D	14

QUESTION 11

Answer	Points
A	0
B	2
C	5
(D)	14

QUESTION 12

Answer	Points
A	25
B	75
C	100
D	100
E	100
F	75
G	75
H	100
I	100
J	0

QUESTION 13

Answer	Points
A	0
B	2
C	5
D	7
E	14

12. **Please select all of the medical conditions that you have or have had in the past.**

a. High blood pressure

b. Gestational diabetes

c. Borderline diabetes or pre-diabetes

d. Diabetes Type II

e. Polycystic ovarian syndrome (PCOS)

f. High triglycerides

g. Low HDL or "good" cholesterol

h. Fatty liver

i. Metabolic Syndrome

j. none

13. **What is your age?**

a. Under 25

b. 26 to 34

c. 35 to 47

d. 48 to 58

e. Over 58

Your MD Factor Quiz Results

It's time to calculate your quiz results. Once you determine your score and know if you have the **MD Factor**, I will give you the steps you need to take to correct your underlying metabolic issues.

The **MD Factor** is caused by changes in how your body is able to use the nutrients in your food. Even if you have not gained a significant amount of weight, your metabolism may no longer be acting the way it used to.

Remember, the **MD Factor** can occur:

✔ When you gain belly weight for any reason, your metabolism changes.

✔ When you have hormonal changes, your metabolism changes.

✔ As you age, your metabolism changes.

Calculate Your Quiz Score

Write in the total point value for each of your answers below.

Part 1	points	Part 2	points	Part 3	points	
Question 1		Question 4		Question 9		
Question 2		Question 5		Question 10		
Question 3		Question 6		Question 11		
		Question 7		Question 12		
		Question 8		Question 13		**Your Total Score**
Part I Total	7	Part 2 Total	10	Part 3 Total	128	143

What Does Your Score Mean?

Your Total
Score

☐

0—19   *Congratulations!* It is unlikely that you have the **MD Factor**. I recommend that you review the **MD Factor** Action Plan and, if you have not already, incorporate my recommended healthy eating plan into your lifestyle.

20—37   Your quiz shows that you are borderline for the **MD Factor**. This means you are in the process of developing the **MD Factor**. This is a great opportunity to make a lasting change now for your health and wellness before you further develop weight or health issues that can accompany the **MD Factor**.

38—77   Your quiz shows that you have the **MD Factor**. You now have an amazing opportunity to follow the **MD Factor** Action Plan, where you will learn the specific way to feed and retrain your body so that you are able to get the best out of your metabolism.

78+   You have a very strong **MD Factor**. I highly recommend following the **MD Factor** Action Plan so that you can restore your metabolism and correct your metabolism dysfunction.

Take the Next Steps to Create a Healthy Future

You now join the thousands who have taken the **MD Factor** Quiz. Whether you score with a low incidence of the **MD Factor** or have a strong **MD Factor**, you have the power to create a healthy future. I will provide you with the power to feed and retrain your body so that you get the best out of your metabolism. You'll see how to do just that with the **MD Factor** Action Plan.

Well-Being & Metabolism Correction Quiz

Check back weekly to take this quiz and track improvement in your well-being and metabolism.

Take this quiz to assess your current well-being and metabolism results. Write this number down. Then, as you begin the **MD Factor** Action Plan, go back and reference this number to track your improvement.

How satisfied are you?

Answer on a scale from 1–7, with 1 being very dissatisfied and 7 being very satisfied.

A. Your weight and physical appearance   (1) 2 3 4 5 6 7

B. Your health   1 2 3 4 5 6 (7)

C. Your energy level   1 2 3 4 5 6 (7)

D. Your ability to focus on tasks   1 2 3 4 (5) 6 7

E. Your sleep   1 2 3 4 (5) 6 7

F. Your hunger level being appropriate   1 2 (3) 4 (5̶) 6 7

G. Your willpower   1 2 (3) 4 5 6 7

As you answer on a scale from 1–7, you will see that if you selected a lower number, this shows an opportunity area for you to be in better health. As you progress through the **MD Factor** Action Plan, check back weekly to take this quiz and track improvement in your well-being and metabolism. As your health improves, you will see an increase in your overall wellness score.

Meet Jennifer, Steve, and Michelle

Jennifer's Story

Jennifer is thirty-two, 5'5", and 230 pounds.
She has the MD Factor due to her weight.

"I wasn't super thin as a teenager, but I wasn't overweight, either. I would say I was solid. I was on my high school softball team and was pretty active.

When I went away to college, I gained the freshman fifteen—actually, it was more like the freshman twenty. I was busy with my classes and worked part time, too. I know I ate too much pizza late at night, and I did drink alcohol, sometimes too much. I went to the gym on and off, but when I graduated I was thirty pounds overweight, at 160. I would love to be back at that weight now.

I got a job with a twenty-five-minute commute, and it was hard to find the time to exercise. I also got into the habit of ordering in or going out for lunch almost every day. Looking back at it now, I realize I was not eating a lot of vegetables. It was more like burgers, sandwiches and chips, pizza—easy, quick food.

I decided enough was enough when my weight climbed to 173. I joined a support group with a friend from work and was able to lose eighteen pounds. She and I walked at lunchtime and brought our own meals to work, and I started cooking more. I am not a fast loser and after six months stopped losing weight. I got to 155, which was not as low as I wanted, but it was better than where I'd been.

I met my husband, Rob, when I was twenty-six, and we married two years later. I tried to lose some more before the wedding, but I think I was actually back to 160. Rob is a big guy; he played football in high school, and he loves to eat. I do, too, and I started to follow his eating habits. You do that when you're married.

I got pregnant pretty soon after our first anniversary. We were thrilled. I felt great during my pregnancy, but my doctor was

"It is so frustrating. I know I'm not perfect, but after a year of dieting on my own, I've lost only three pounds, and I'm tired and hungry all the time."

concerned I was gaining too much weight. After I'd gained almost forty pounds, I was tested for gestational [pregnancy-related] diabetes. The test showed I had it, but luckily I didn't need to take insulin. I had to meet with a dietitian, who told me to eat less bread and sugars and eat more vegetables and protein. I delivered my son two weeks early, which was probably a good thing, as he was already nine pounds. I weighed 215 when I delivered him, but I have to admit I stopped looking at the scale when I passed the 200 mark.

My son, Brandon, was a very colicky baby. I got very little sleep, especially as I had to go back to work after eight weeks. The next two years were a blur. Rob and I both work, but due to our schedules, I had to get Brandon fed, dressed, and off to day care before I got to work. I never had time to eat breakfast, but I grabbed a Diet Coke for the caffeine. I'm not hungry in the morning anyway. I fell into my old pattern of going out to lunch and getting takeout for meals at home, too. It was really hard to shop and cook when I was so completely exhausted.

I lost fifteen pounds after Brandon's birth, but I gained that back and then some. So last year, when I hit 233, I started the support group online. I started eating some fruit or cereal in the morning, but that actually makes me hungrier. I make a turkey sandwich on two slices of really thinly sliced bread and bring pretzels and fruit for lunch. But I'm so hungry for dinner that it's nearly impossible to take the time to make a healthful meal like grilled chicken and salad and vegetables. Some days I do it, but others I end up eating crackers and cheese or pretzels or grapes while trying to get dinner on. Other days I just give in and order Chinese food or pizza.

Even though I am so tired, I have been forcing myself to go to the gym and do the treadmill, usually on Saturdays and one night during the week when Rob gets home earlier.

It is so frustrating. I know I'm not perfect, but after a year of dieting on my own, I've lost only three pounds, and I'm tired and hungry all the time. Some days I just don't even bother to diet because it doesn't seem to make a difference anyway. I'm very worried because I want to have another child in a few years and I'm afraid I won't be healthy enough to do so. What is wrong with me and my metabolism? I was able to lose weight before by following the same plan I am following now, but it's stopped working. I'm only thirty-two. If I don't get a handle on this now, I'm not going to be able to keep up with my son as he runs around. Please help me."

Steve's Story

Steve is forty-five, 5'10", and 220 pounds.
He has the MD Factor due to getting older.

"It's been hard for me to get my weight under control for the past few years. I was an athlete in high school, and I've always liked to exercise. I'd prefer to play basketball or softball, but that can be hard to coordinate with work and family life, so I've been going to the gym for the past fifteen years at least. I'd been able to eat what I wanted as long as I was consistent with doing the treadmill twice a week and lifting weights three days a week for at least an hour. On weekends I am busy with my kids; I'm my seven-year-old son's soccer coach on Saturdays. It is not a heavy workout, but there's a lot of running!

But even though my exercise routine is the same and my eating habits haven't changed, my weight has been creeping up over the past few years, especially once I turned forty. It was only a few pounds a year, but over the past four years it's been cumulative, and now I am twenty-five pounds heavier than I was in my thirties.

My wife makes healthy meals at least three times a week, like chicken with vegetables or pasta with red sauce, and I cook steak on the grill once a week. We try to do one date night a week where my wife and I go to a restaurant and get a break from the kids. Friday night is pizza night, and one night is usually leftovers. My lunches are pretty healthy, too. I eat lunch out, but usually I order a salad with chicken or fish or a sandwich. I do eat the chips or whatever comes with it, but again, that is nothing new. I've never been much of a breakfast eater—usually just coffee after the gym.

What's annoying is that in my thirties, if I gained a few pounds, I'd just cut down by skipping lunch a few days a week or eating less at dinner and I could easily lose three to five pounds in a few days. That doesn't happen anymore. I guess because I'm older, right?

I've also gotten a gut like I see a lot of men in their forties and fifties have. That bothers me a lot because

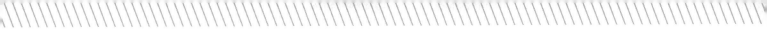

I still work out and feel I'm athletic. I had a physical when I turned forty-two and my doctor told me my cholesterol wasn't great and my blood pressure was creeping up. Cholesterol medicine doesn't work for what I have, and he told me to start exercising. That was aggravating, as I already exercise five days a week. So then he told me to cut out soda and junk food. I really haven't had fast food since before I was married, and I stopped drinking Cokes years ago.

I need to get this weight under control. My wife is worried, and so am I, as my father, who'd always done physical work but never any kind of exercise regimen, had a heart attack in his early fifties. He survived it, but it really affected him—he was never as active again and always seemed short of breath. He also had a big gut at the same age I am now, and I thought it was because he didn't work out. I don't want to have a heart attack. And I want my energy level to get back to what it was. I'm more tired than I used to be, and I don't want to be the kind of dad who's too pooped to run after his kids!"

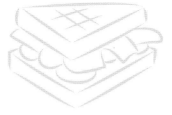

"I could easily lose three to five pounds in a few days. That doesn't happen anymore. I guess because I'm older, right?"

Michelle's Story

Michelle is fifty-four, 5'4" tall, and weighs 145 pounds. **She has the MD Factor because of hormonal changes.**

"I know my metabolism has changed. Ever since I turned forty-nine the weight has been piling on. I was 115 lbs. when I graduated from high school and have been 118 lbs. for all of my adult life until recently. I've never had a weight problem before, and now I have all this belly fat and cellulite. I can't stand it!

I was really thin as a child and my mother was so worried about me that she took me to the doctor. He said I was fine but she should give me milkshakes and let me eat what I wanted. I was always very active, and I still am; I don't stop all day. I am a type A personality and always have a lot going on. I am on the computer and phone at work—I'm in sales and have a great career—but I also walk around my office a lot. I have to admit, recently I've been having energy slumps around 3:00 p.m. and need to grab coffee. I also fantasize about a quick nap but never take one. I never had those energy slumps before.

I have always eaten whatever I wanted, and I never dieted. When I travel and meet with clients, I eat out a lot—the portions are too big, but I never finish my meal. I prefer healthier foods. I avoid fried foods except french fries, and I love vegetables. I am a big fan of ethnic foods and have been for years. I do like my wine, though, and I usually have two glasses of wine each night, as it helps me relax.

I wouldn't say I was a heavy exerciser like some of my friends who are runners, but I walked my dogs at least a mile a day when I was home, and I played tennis if I got a chance, just for fun.

When I was forty-nine, my skirts and my pants seemed to be getting tight. It was odd, because nothing had changed with my diet and exercise. The first few times I noticed it, I actually thought the dry cleaner had shrunk some of my clothes! I also realized that I wasn't sleeping as well, either. Some nights I'd wake up at two

"I really feel like my body has let me down. Menopause is awful, and the worst part is all the weight gain."

o'clock and be too alert to go back to sleep. Other nights I had some night sweats, so I saw my doctor, who told me I was going through perimenopause and that I could take hormones if I wanted. My mother had breast cancer in her early fifties, so I was not too excited about the prospect of the hormones. I could live with the hot flashes. What I can't live with is the weight gain.

I'd never dieted before, but I cut down on everything. I decreased my portions and ate less pasta, because my friends who are always dieting told me it puts weight on. I wasn't a huge dessert eater, but I cut out desserts and other sweets. What is weird is that I noticed I had been craving sweets more in the past few years, and I don't remember ever craving them before.

Despite that, I gained ten pounds in a year. I saw my doctor again and told him to check my thyroid and anything else, but all my numbers were normal. He said that I needed to exercise more and eat less, which wasn't helpful at all! Still, I started working with a personal trainer. He works me out, hard. We lift weights and do cardio three times a week. I am so sore after the workouts. I know I am getting stronger and more toned, but I didn't lose any weight, so I added two more days of cardio during the weeks I don't travel. My appearance is very important for the impression I need to make at work.

I can't believe my weight hasn't budged. I'm eating so much less than I ever did before and exercising so much more, and I still have not lost any weight. In fact, I'm gaining. I even cut down on wine and then stopped it altogether for two weeks, but it made no difference in my weight, so I started having wine again.

Despite all my hard work, I've still gained more than twenty pounds in the last five years. I went back to my doctor and he told me my cholesterol was high and I should start medicine for it. He also told me my blood pressure was creeping up. I told him I wanted more tests to find out why I can't lose weight, and he referred me to you. I don't want to take medicine and I can't stand this weight. I love clothes and have a closet full of expensive designer clothes I can't wear. I used to enjoy shopping, but now it's too depressing. I am not even comfortable in my underwear because so much of my weight is in my belly area. I refuse to buy larger sizes!

I could understand this weight gain if I was eating all day and not exercising, but I'm not. I really feel like my body has let me down. Menopause is awful, and the worst part is all the weight gain."

Does any of this sound familiar to you? Read on to find out what I recommended to Jennifer, Steve, and Michelle. And at the end of the book, on pages 183–185, you'll see what happened for them once they started following the **MD Factor** Action Plan.

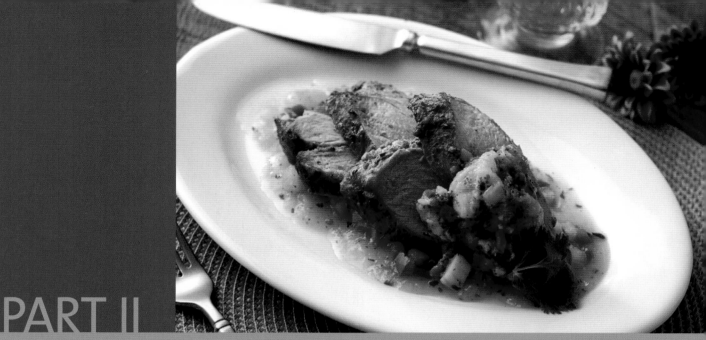

Jerk pork tenderloin

PART II

UNDERSTANDING THE MD FACTOR

CHAPTER 2

The MD Factor = Metabolism Dysfunction

If counting calories and sweating it out during intense workouts can't melt those pounds anymore—if you're doing everything you've been told to do in order to lose weight but nothing's working—stop blaming yourself. Something isn't right with how your body is functioning. There has to be an underlying factor making your body resist what should be a steady weight loss, because our bodies are not stubborn without a good reason!

The reason, of course, is the **MD Factor**. When you have it, your metabolism is out of whack. It's not what it used to be because it's *dysfunctional*.

Not only that, but the **MD Factor** means that your metabolism loves to store fat and hates to let go of it. This means you can gain weight even when you're meticulously watching what you eat. Just what you needed, right?

What Causes the **MD Factor?**

The overwhelming majority of my patients who've put up a valiant yet fruitless battle against the bulge have insulin resistance—what I'm calling the **MD Factor**. It's a very common metabolic condition, but because it flies under the radar, it can be overlooked, even by medical professionals.

The **MD Factor** simply means that your cells are resistant to the action of insulin, a hormone produced by your pancreas that regulates how your cells metabolize energy. (I'll explain *why* the **MD Factor** happens in Chapter 3.) The sensitivity of your cells to insulin is crucial for weight management, as insulin directs fuel to your cells so that they can have energy and perform all the day-to-day cellular functions to keep you healthy and moving.

In your body, insulin acts like a key that unlocks the door to your cells—the medical term for this door is "glucose portal"—and allows glucose (sugar) to get inside. Your body likes to use glucose for its metabolic needs, because it's very efficient and produces a lot of energy.

But if you have the **MD Factor**, the insulin key doesn't fit into the lock of the glucose portal anymore. The cell remains shut, even if it's desperate for fuel. And when these cells become starved for fuel, you already know what happens. Your ravenously hungry cells send signals to your brain, telling you to do whatever you can to get sugar into your body—pronto!

To make matters worse for those with the **MD Factor**, there is the problem of what to do with all that glucose that remains *outside* your cells. Your body is pretty smart about its needs for fuel, especially because human beings evolved when food was not as easy as it is to obtain now. So your body says, "Hey, I'm not going to waste all this perfectly good

Do You Know What Fat Really Is?

What few dieters know is that fat is primarily composed of lots of glucose molecules, with some additional biochemical adjustments, linked together in a nice, usable package. When your body does need fuel and goes to use this stored fat, it breaks down the links between these glucose molecules and delivers them to your bloodstream.

In other words, when your body is burning fat, it's really burning sugar!

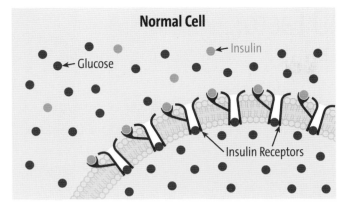

Normal Cell

Glucose

Insulin

Insulin Receptors

Healthy amounts of glucose inside the cell will fuel the cell. Also note there are normal glucose and insulin levels outside the cell.

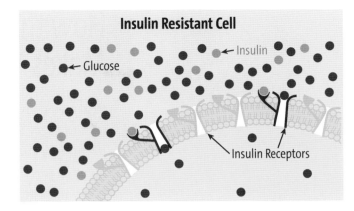

Insulin Resistant Cell

Glucose

Insulin

Insulin Receptors

Here there is so little glucose or energy inside the cell, the cell is starving. Outside the cell, there are higher glucose and insulin levels. This extra glucose will be converted to fat.

fuel. I might be starving tomorrow! I'm going to store it, just in case. Even better, I'm not going to store it as sugar—I'm going to stash it away as plump, juicy *fat*."

What's the Difference between the **MD Factor** and Metabolic Syndrome?

Thirty percent of all American adults, including 47 percent of those over the age of fifty, have such an advanced case of MD Factor that it has a clinical name: metabolic syndrome. Having metabolic syndrome drastically increases your likelihood of developing diabetes, heart disease, stroke, or cancer. Many of my patients do have metabolic syndrome, but they had no idea that their metabolism was changing so drastically. All they knew is that they kept on gaining weight, first in their bellies and then all over their bodies, and nothing they did reversed it. Fortunately, the MD Factor Action Plan can help cure metabolic syndrome.

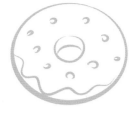

How the **MD Factor** Makes You Feel

When you have the **MD Factor**, your pancreas produces lots of extra insulin to try to get glucose into cells that are no longer as sensitive to the hormone as they used to be. (Many of my patients have insulin levels as much as three to ten times higher than normal.) Much the way a battering ram will eventually break down the door to the castle, producing excess insulin means that at least some of the glucose in your bloodstream will get into those starving cells. But when the glucose finally reaches its destination, your blood sugar will plummet. This is called low blood sugar, or hypoglycemia, and it can trigger a number of symptoms, including cravings, lack of energy, mental fogginess, shakiness, and trouble sleeping.

Craving Sweets? Your Cells Are Starving for Sugar

The most common symptom of the **MD Factor** is a craving for sweets or carbohydrates. Steve is a good example. He never ate breakfast. He'd have a large black coffee, and that kept him going all morning. By lunchtime, he still wasn't very hungry, but he'd have something small, like a salad with some chicken. And then he'd be so tired he had to take a short nap (which wasn't very refreshing). When he woke up, he was desperately craving either something soft and sweet, such as chocolate chip cookies, or something crunchy and salty, maybe potato chips or pretzels. He knew this wasn't healthful, but he couldn't break the cycle because he just couldn't bear the thought of eating any breakfast.

Same with Jennifer. *"I know I'm supposed to eat breakfast, so I force myself to have some whole-grain cereal or fruit and a piece of whole-wheat toast, but when I do this, I'm so ravenously hungry by ten in the morning that I practically keel over. So then I gobble up the only kind of food available at work, usually doughnuts. I've tried this over and over, and it always happens. Being five times hungrier after what's supposedly a healthful breakfast and then chowing down on doughnuts isn't helping me lose weight!"*

Steve and Jennifer have a typical **MD Factor** pattern. When their cells were unable to get the glucose they needed, they responded with a vengeance. Mike's post-lunchtime brain was screaming, *"Naptime now!"* And when he woke up, his midafternoon brain was shrieking, *"Feed me now!"* Jennifer's insulin-driven appetite didn't even carry her from breakfast to lunch—she just had to eat.

Michelle was also worried. *"I've never been a big sweets eater,"* she told me, *"but now I feel like I physically crave them. I want to lose weight and eat sensibly, but then I go out and buy a candy bar an hour after lunch, or turn the cupboard inside out a few hours after dinner searching for something sweet. I haven't been doing this my whole life. This is new. Something has changed, and it's driving me crazy!"*

Steve unwittingly blamed himself for his eating pattern because he had no idea what the **MD Factor** was doing to him. *"I normally eat a healthy-size portion for lunch or dinner—more than enough food—but I still want sweet or starchy afterward,"* he explained. *"It must be all in my head, or because I'm stressed or something. I mean, I'm an intelligent person, and I know that when I've eaten seven or eight hundred calories during a meal, it should be enough. But I just keep going, and then I find myself eating things that I'd promised myself I wouldn't eat. And then I start over the next day with the best intentions, only to blow it by dinner. Why do I keep eating sugar and junk food when my goal is to lose weight? I know better and want better for myself, but obviously I can't do it on my own."*

Stories like these are incredibly common. Steve, Jennifer, and Michelle all crave the very foods they know they shouldn't eat because their starving cells send distress signals to other cells, which in turn respond by producing hormones, chemical messages to their brains that compel them to eat the kind of starchy carbohydrates that can quickly deliver sugar into their bloodstreams.

This sets up the devastating **MD Factor** cycle. Your cells scream and shout at you to eat carbs and sugars, but because you have the **MD Factor**, all that glucose *still* can't get into your starving cells, so it gets stored as fat . . . plus, you're still hungry! So you eat more carbs and sugars and pack on the pounds. To make things worse, at the same time, your metabolic rate begins to drop because when your body doesn't get the right amount of fuel it needs on a regular basis, it tries to conserve as much energy as possible. The result is that your body needs fewer calories, so even eating the same amount you used to eat will result in weight gain.

Low Energy Level?
The Cause Is Low Blood Sugar

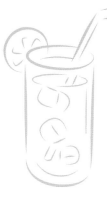

Does this sound familiar? Your energy level plummets several hours after you eat, especially in the afternoon. You can get so tired after eating that you absolutely need to lie down and take a nap. You might also feel weak, dizzy, or shaky if you're late for your usual mealtime, or several hours after a meal that was particularly high in sugar or carbohydrates. Your concentration can be poor. People tend to describe this as having a "fuzzy head" or "brain fog."

"I have a really big dip in energy around three in the afternoon," Jennifer told me. *"I feel weak and tired and it's really hard to stay focused at work. When this happens on weekends, I normally take a nap, but I can't do that during the week. So I eat a little something, which helps me come out of it. But the snacking means that I'm gaining weight. I try to stop doing this—sometimes I'll skip lunch and just drink lots of water—but when I do that, I'm like a wild woman when I get home. I'll eat anything that won't eat me first! I'll power through an entire bag of chips or a pack of crackers with a big hunk of cheese. I'll keep eating this kind of stuff when I'm making dinner. If I'm cooking a nice meal and it'll be ready in twenty minutes, I swear I can't wait. Do I have diabetes or something?"*

Luckily, Jennifer does not have diabetes, but her "something" is the **MD Factor**. Her blood sugar fluctuations are sharpening her appetite. And people with the **MD Factor** tend to eat very fast, scarfing down a huge amount of calories in only a few minutes. The reason they do this is because hypoglycemia, or low blood sugar, is a threat to the proper functioning of the body.

Bear in mind, though, that this type of hypoglycemia is not the same as what diabetics live with. Anyone who must inject insulin needs to be meticulous about it, as their blood sugar levels can decline drastically afterward, causing them to faint, have a convulsion, or even die. This is truly life threatening—but it is *not* the type of low blood sugar the

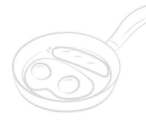

MD Factor causes. However, people with the **MD Factor** do experience relative drops in blood sugar, and these can make you feel awful.

Rarely Hungry in the Morning? You're Producing Too Much Insulin

If you have the **MD Factor**, you may not be hungry when you wake up, and you may find it hard to eat breakfast or sometimes even lunch. Instead, you start getting intense hunger pangs in the middle of the afternoon, and when you do eat, you don't seem to feel full.

When you have the **MD Factor**, you'll usually wake up with a higher than normal level of insulin circulating in your blood, trying to open up those locked cells. This is not normal, because usually insulin is released after you eat. So if you haven't eaten for eight hours, you should have a very low level of insulin in your blood. These higher insulin levels explain why you aren't hungry at all.

When you have too much insulin and then eat carbohydrate-rich foods for breakfast, look out! This is what happens:

✔ Sugar gets absorbed into your bloodstream.

✔ Your blood sugar spikes and then drops rapidly because the extra insulin is battering at the glucose portals of your cells, trying to get that sugar out of your bloodstream and into the starving cells.

✔ Your body perceives the dropping blood sugar, so it sends distress signals of hunger, telling you to eat so that your blood sugar level will go back up.

For example, if you have the **MD Factor**, when you eat an allegedly healthful breakfast, such as whole-grain cereal, fruit, or a bagel with a tiny bit of butter, all these carbs are rapidly processed since your insulin level is already high to begin with. The result is that your blood sugar falls just as rapidly, even dipping below normal within a short span of time, so you get hungry again!

If, on the other hand, you do have normal insulin levels in the morning, or if you have the **MD Factor** and your breakfast contains less carbohydrate and sugar—which is what you'll eat on the **MD Factor** Action Plan—then this process is much more gradual and controlled.

A normal blood sugar response after a meal should be like riding a bike over gently sloping hills, up and down, slowly and evenly, over the course of several hours. With the **MD Factor**, however, these drops are like sharp jags and spikes—and you're going to fall off your bike!

This graph shows what happens when someone with the **MD Factor** eats. GL, or glycemic load, refers to how much your blood glucose rises after a meal. A high-glycemic-load meal would be cereal, toast, and juice (all sugar and carbohydrates). A low-glycemic-load meal would be eggs scrambled with peppers, onions, and Canadian bacon (mostly protein).

When blood sugar falls rapidly, the *rate* of the fall is what triggers many of the **MD Factor** symptoms. Look at the graph again, and you'll see that with the high-glycemic-load meal, blood sugar dips below normal about an hour and forty-five minutes after eating. Because your body doesn't know why your blood sugar is falling or how low it will go, it panics, releasing the stress hormone epinephrine. This is what causes that shaky, anxious feeling where you just have to eat.

These jittery symptoms won't happen if you eat the right kind of breakfast, one that provides your body with the nutrition that it needs.

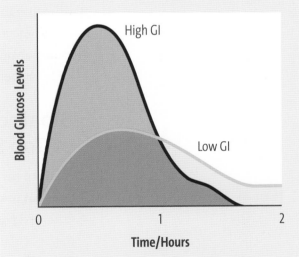

In the graph above, the amount of carbohydrate in the reference and test food must be the same.

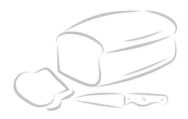

Got Brain Fog? It's the Result of Too Much Insulin

After having a meal that is high in carbohydrates, such as pasta with a side of garlic bread, you feel foggy and exhausted, right? Or do you feel fuzzy, blah, spaced out, or sluggish after you eat something with a lot of sugar? Do you find it hard to concentrate or be precise? Does your mind wander while you get nothing accomplished at your desk?

This is not a normal metabolic response to a carbohydrate meal. But if you have the **MD Factor**, it is what you can expect. All that insulin has a direct effect on the water and electrolyte levels in your brain. Electrolytes such as sodium, potassium, and magnesium are in careful balance inside and outside all our cells. Excess insulin causes these electrolytes to enter the brain cells in a slightly increased amount, and then water follows these electrolytes in. The result is a slight swelling of your brain tissues, so your thinking can't be as fast or crisp as it should be. A study published in the *Journal of Holistic Medicine* proved that susceptible people (such as those with the **MD Factor**) showed changes to their brain wave signals and communication after eating a high-carbohydrate meal.

Bloated? Another Result of Too Much Insulin

Many of my patients complain that their faces, arms, and legs are puffy and that their abdomens are bloated. This is likely related to the same fluid and electrolyte change that's triggered by too much insulin. Sodium, in particular, causes puffiness and bloat, which is why your jeans can feel extra tight after a salty meal. (When that happens, drinking lots of water to rehydrate your tissues and flush the extra sodium out of your system is the best solution.)

Fortunately, when you start the **MD Factor** Action Plan, you should see a drop in water weight along with body fat the very first week. The longer you stay on the plan, the less likely it is that any puffiness or bloat will return.

Trouble Sleeping? Low Blood Sugar Is the Culprit

A common symptom of the **MD Factor** is that you sleep poorly, often waking in the wee hours—and feeling wide awake when that happens.

"Usually I have no trouble falling asleep," Michelle said, *"but just a few hours later I wake up. Not just wake up—I'm wide awake, as if I'd already had seven hours of sleep when I really only had three. I'll toss and turn, or else I'll give up and get up to do some work. I feel okay then, but then by 5:00 p.m. the next day I'm totally wiped out. I notice this happens even more often if I have a few glasses of wine in the evening."*

Michelle's **MD Factor** causes her blood sugar to drop, and alcohol makes it worse. That's because alcohol first raises your blood sugar and then lowers it after an insulin release. Even two glasses of wine can be enough to cause you to wake up from a sound sleep in the middle of the night. This is an important part of managing the **MD Factor**, so if you drink alcohol regularly, Chapter 9 is a must-read.

It's a lot easier to lose weight if you aren't constantly hungry, tired, cranky, weak, and craving sugar!

Bottom Line

The **MD Factor** responds incredibly quickly to the right kind of eating plan, which is why Part III will help you right away. Usually it takes only a week or two on the Action Plan before your symptoms start to lessen and then disappear entirely. It's a lot easier to lose weight if you aren't constantly hungry, tired, cranky, weak, and craving sugar!

CHAPTER 3

Triggers for the MD Factor

When you have the **MD Factor**, it's easy to feel defeated, especially when you're trying your hardest to lose weight and not seeing any results. But you are not alone. By now, it should be very clear just how common the **MD Factor** really is.

What Triggers the **MD Factor?**

The **MD Factor** doesn't develop overnight. There are many reasons for it, and your particular situation may be caused by a combination of the following:

Genetic Predisposition

This is the one reason you have no control over, because genetic factors are inherited from your parents. To see how genetic factors affected me and my family members, go to Appendix D, where you can read about new genetic testing that can reveal more information about your personal predisposition to the **MD Factor**.

Some people are lucky and don't have genes that make it likely they'll have the **MD Factor**. Chances are good, however, that you were born with a tendency to have cells that don't respond particularly well to insulin. And if there's a strong family history of diabetes, particularly from your parents, you are at high risk. In my practice, I've treated children, teens, and young adults who have the **MD Factor** thanks to their genes and certain lifestyle factors that cause these genes to become active.

Your genes also regulate where your body stores fat. Take a look: If you are a pear shape, you tend to store your weight in your hips, buttocks, and thighs. If, however, you're an apple shape, you'll store fat in your abdominal area, as well as your sides and lower back. Many of my patients tell me that everyone in their families, even the thin ones, have a bit of a pooch. "I have the Smith family belly!" they say.

Belly or Visceral Fat

If you have a tendency to store fat in your abdominal area, when you gain weight your body adds significantly to the thin layer of protective and

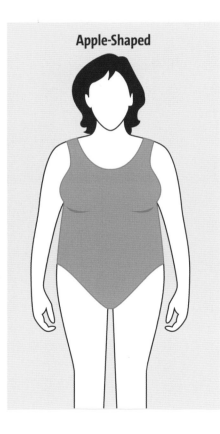

Apple-Shaped

cushioning fat tissue that normally surrounds your vital organs, such as your liver. This is called visceral fat.

Extra visceral fat hinders organs from functioning properly, especially your liver, which has to sift through a lot of fat tissue to do its job, which is ridding your body of toxins. In addition, as the **MD Factor** progresses, fat actually gets deposited *inside* your organs. When this happens to your liver, its cells now have fat stored in them (this is called fatty liver).

Visceral fat puts you at a higher risk for developing the **MD Factor**. In addition, it increases bad cholesterol while lowering good cholesterol levels. It also increases levels of inflammatory hormones, which are significant contributing factors for heart disease.

And since men deposit fat in the abdomen whenever they gain weight, while women prior to menopause usually deposit extra weight in their hips and thighs, this explains why men often develop heart disease ten to twenty years before women do. After menopause, however, when women start depositing visceral fat in their abdomen, their rate of heart disease catches up to or even surpasses that of men.

People of different ethnicities have a greater or lesser likelihood of developing more or less visceral fat. CAT scans used by researchers to see where body fat is stored show that people of East Asian or South Asian descent tend to have the largest amounts of visceral fat. This is one reason that diabetes is so prevalent in China, India, and Chinese and Indian communities elsewhere in the world. There has been scientific discussion as to whether people of Asian descent need to be considered overweight at a much lighter weight than Caucasians because an Asian person is likely to carry almost all of his or her excess weight in the dangerous visceral fat location.

People of Hispanic descent and Native Americans also have higher levels of visceral fat and a higher risk of developing the **MD Factor** than Caucasian Americans. A study published a few years ago in the *Journal*

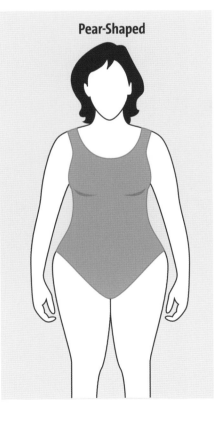

Pear-Shaped

Very few of us can eat the same way at thirty as we did at ten, or can eat at fifty what we ate at thirty.

of the American Medical Association forecast that of American girls of Hispanic descent born in the year 2000, a full 50 percent will develop type 2 diabetes, which is very alarming. And as you know, type 2 diabetes occurs when the **MD Factor** is not treated and corrected.

Daily Stress

The daily stress of life in the twenty-first century can take a toll on your waistline, making you gain weight either gradually or suddenly. Perhaps you have a new job or a new baby, your kids are having trouble in school or you need to move, or your parents become ill or a beloved family member dies. Maybe you're just too busy to find the time to exercise and cook healthful food the way you used to, so you have nutritional deficiencies. Or you might finally stop smoking. In all of these cases, the weight can creep up before you know it.

Normal Aging

As we grow older, our hormones gradually decline. This is a natural, normal process that happens to everyone. Women lose estrogen and progesterone, men lose testosterone, and both lose human growth hormone. These declining hormonal levels also affect muscle mass. Add in a more sedentary lifestyle, and here comes the **MD Factor**. There are, after all, very few of us who can eat the same way at thirty as we did at ten, or who can eat at fifty what we ate at thirty.

That means that as you age, your changing body needs you to change your eating habits, too. Normal aging, when combined with other risk factors, contributes substantially to the development of the **MD Factor**. Doctors have known for years that the risk of diabetes increases as people get older, and a specific medical study conducted more than thirty years ago concluded that carbohydrate intolerance develops as a part of the normal aging process. But what was not clear at the time, nor to many in the medical community still today, is the reason the **MD Factor** increases with age.

Many people already feel a sense of anxiety regarding the aging process, but to be blunt, aging in a healthy manner is far better than the alternative, which is an early death. If we are to avoid weight gain, diabetes, and other related medical problems as we age, we need to become more aware of the **MD Factor** and eat and exercise in such a way as to minimize its effects.

Often experts will say things like, "The only reason that people gain weight as they age is that they are eating more calories than they need. They're simply not burning as many calories as they are taking in." However, this calories-in/calories-out logic is simply not how the human body works. This simplistic approach to weight gain with age ignores the important metabolic fact that the **MD Factor** is a very real condition that plays a large role in the process.

What researchers uncovered at least thirty years ago was that when people of a normal weight are compared by age, the amount of insulin their bodies secrete after a test meal of sugar increases with age. This study found that normal weight people in their sixties secreted far more insulin and also had higher blood sugar levels after consuming the test meal than did people in their thirties.

There is also a loss of muscle mass that comes with aging. The conventional thought has always been that this loss of muscle contributes to the risk factors that produce the **MD Factor**. While this is true, the process is a whole lot more complicated. In fact, the **MD Factor** also directly *causes* a loss of muscle tissue. As our cells burn energy sources as part of the metabolic process, waste by-products called reactive oxygen species build up and damage the mitochondria, which are the tiny components of our cells that are responsible for creating energy.

It is far easier to prevent weight gain than to lose weight. It's easier to lose fifteen pounds than it is to lose thirty.

When mitochondria do not function properly, the food that we eat cannot be metabolized normally. Instead of being burned, fat accumulates in the cells and impairs the function of insulin. With this comes the **MD Factor** and a downward spiral that leads to the breakdown of muscle mass, as well as a decrease in the creation of new muscle.

Unfortunately, those with the **MD Factor** are also destined to experience higher than normal blood sugar levels, which cause even more damage to the cells. This really is a vicious cycle that you must address sooner rather than later. But take heart—studies have shown that a person's amount of body fat affects the **MD Factor** more than age does. This is extremely good news! It means that although you can't slow down time, you *can* control one of the single biggest risk factors for the **MD Factor**: what you eat and when.

One last note about the **MD Factor** and aging. It is never too soon to start working on controlling your weight. I see plenty of people in my practice in their forties who have gained around fifteen pounds that they find very difficult to lose. The reasons they have gained the weight are different for each person, but the end result is the same: they are more likely to develop the **MD Factor**. Sometimes patients who've only gained five or ten pounds tell me that when they've discussed this with their friends, the reaction is often, "Why do you need to see a doctor when you've only gained a few pounds?" When that happens, I tell my patients that they're very smart to be so proactive about their weight gain and that it's always important for everyone to get their metabolism back on track. It is far easier to prevent weight gain than to lose weight. It's easier to lose fifteen pounds than it is to lose thirty.

We will all get older. As we get older, the effect of the **MD Factor** becomes stronger. However, we all have the power to minimize that effect and prevent future medical problems.

Your Medications

Many different medications can contribute to the **MD Factor**. In fact, there are more than 480 drugs with weight gain as a known side effect. This can be a big problem for weight loss when you have a medical condition and you need to take these drugs in order to get healthy or stay healthy, especially when there are no safe or effective substitutions available for them. Sometimes there may be substitutions that might be just as effective, so discuss your alternatives with your doctor and follow the **MD Factor** Action Plan.

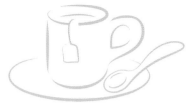

Medications That Often Cause Weight Gain

✔ Antidepressants

✔ Antihistamines

✔ Anti-anxiety medications

✔ Anti-inflammatories (particularly steroids)

✔ Anti-seizure medications

✔ Birth control pills or progesterone injections

✔ Blood pressure medications (such as beta-blockers or diuretics)

✔ Insulin shots

✔ Psychotropic medications (for bipolar disorder or schizophrenia)

Nutritional Deficiencies

When your body doesn't get the right fuel it needs to keep it running smoothly, the **MD Factor** can appear. The most common nutritional deficiency has to do with how much protein you eat and when you eat it. Other common deficiency triggers are a lack of vitamin D, vitamin B12, and magnesium. You'll read much more about protein in Chapter 4 and supplements in Chapter 7, and you can see what blood tests I recommend in Appendix B.

Your Thyroid and Metabolism

If you have many of the symptoms in the list below, you need to have blood work done. Your doctor should look at your levels of T4 (inactive thyroid hormone), T3 (active thyroid hormone), and TSH (thyroid-stimulating hormone); be sure to insist that your physician tests you

Initial Symptoms of Hypothyroidism	Symptoms of Advanced Hypothyroidism
✔ Constipation	✔ Depression and decreasing mental stability
✔ Forgetfulness	✔ Dry, flaky, inelastic skin
✔ High cholesterol	✔ Dry, sparse hair
✔ Menstrual changes (too heavy or very light, too frequent or too infrequent)	✔ Fluid under the eyes
✔ Sensitivity to cold	✔ Hoarseness
✔ Unexplained weight gain	✔ Puffy face, hands, and feet
	✔ Thick, brittle nails
	✔ Upper eyelid droop

for T3, which is often not ordered. Often women, especially after menopause, have a hard time converting T4 into T3 and may show lower T3 levels even with an otherwise normal thyroid blood test profile. Hypothyroidism responds well to treatment with replacement thyroid hormones.

Understanding Why Your Thyroid Is Important

Your body is regulated by different hormones secreted by various glands. Your adrenal glands pump out hormones such as cortisol and adrenaline when you're stressed or frightened. Your thyroid gland pumps out hormones that regulate much of your body's metabolic functions.

Because your thyroid is so crucial to metabolic functioning, many of my patients assume that extra weight means they have low levels of thyroid hormone, or hypothyroidism—which is very common, especially in women over the age of forty—and that fixing this means their metabolism will automatically rev back up and the pounds they've put on will melt away. I wish that were true, but it's usually not. Regaining normal thyroid levels does make you feel better, with improved energy, but unless you address the **MD Factor**, you can still gain weight and unwanted visceral fat.

For Women Only: Menopause

For so many women, the hormonal changes that take place during perimenopause (when the female hormones, estrogen and progesterone, start to decline) and menopause (when menstruation ceases) are no joy. They can cause symptoms that range from mood swings, irritability, foggy thinking, hot flashes, night sweats, dry skin and hair, and lighter or heavier periods to depression, insomnia, low libido, and weight gain. *Especially* weight gain. In fact, the average woman puts on a whopping thirty pounds during menopause. And no, thirty is not a typo!

Many women will do whatever it takes to manage these symptoms, not only to try to lose weight but also to feel better. That leads them to hormone replacement therapy, or HRT. HRT has long been controversial, and it has been more so since a comprehensive trial undertaken by the Women's Health Initiative and published in 2002 shockingly showed that women who took the hormone Prempro, made from synthetic estrogen and progesterone, increased their risk of heart disease, stroke, and breast cancer.

Before that, doctors had thought that estrogen and progesterone protected a woman's heart, based on epidemiological studies showing that women who used HRT lived longer and had less heart disease. Doctors often prescribed HRT with the intention to protect women's hearts from coronary artery disease, as well as their bones from osteoporosis. Yes, there was a health risk trade-off, with a slight increase in the risk of breast cancer and uterine cancer in HRT users, but for many women, the benefit of improved bone and heart health made sense, as more women die of heart disease or hip fractures than from breast cancer.

Since this study came out, however, HRT has been prescribed much less frequently, and only if symptoms are so severe as to affect a woman's quality of life. If you're considering HRT, discuss the risks and benefits with your physician so you can make an informed decision. Typically, HRT is prescribed in the lowest possible dose for the shortest possible time.

But here's what you need to know about HRT and weight gain: the average menopausal woman will gain that thirty pounds whether she chooses to use HRT or not! Often those on HRT find that they don't gain weight at first, but after several years they realize that the pounds are slowly piling on. And for all women, on HRT or not, the distribution of their fat shifts; waists get thicker while hips and thighs seem somewhat smaller. This means that even if you haven't gained a pound, your fat distribution is likely to change. (Hello, pooch!) Eventually, though, the weight is stored everywhere. In other words, replacing female hormones doesn't prevent the **MD Factor**.

So what is estrogen's role in the **MD Factor**? Scientists studying how estrogen receptors function in the hypothalamus—the part of the brain controlling body temperature, hunger, thirst, fatigue, and sleep cycles—finally cracked the code. The hypothalamus is basically a master switch to control food intake, energy expenditure, and body fat distribution. When these scientists disabled the estrogen receptors in lab rats (which are used in studies like these because their physiology is similar to that of

Hot Flashes and Hypoglycemia

When you're going through perimenopause or menopause, one of the easiest ways to trigger a hot flash is to eat a high-carbohydrate meal—say, bread, a large bowl of pasta, a glass or two of wine, and a sugary dessert. Even if you're on HRT, this kind of eating will likely get you all hot and bothered!

Hot flashes are a misreading by the temperature control of your body, located in the hypothalamus, and hypoglycemia plays a huge role in triggering them. Keeping blood sugar levels stable is, as you know, a delicate balance. After you eat, your body absorbs sugar into your bloodstream; blood sugar rises steadily after a meal and begins to fall as your cells take in sugar. When levels drop a few hours after a high-carbohydrate meal, your body essentially panics in order to prevent levels from dropping too low. If you already have naturally low amounts of estrogen, the hypothalamus can be activated more easily. The result is that you feel hot and flushed, which is followed by a shaky clamminess once your body settles down.

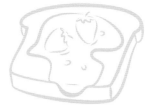

humans), the animals immediately began to eat more food, display lower energy levels and a lower metabolic rate (they acted sluggish), and pack on pounds in the worst place possible (visceral fat in their abdomen). Even when they were fed the same amount of food, they still gained a substantial amount of weight!

What I found stunning about these conclusions is that the weight issues women experience with menopause have not changed, even with the massive overhaul in how menopause has been treated. Before the Women's Health Initiative study was published in 2002, most of my perimenopausal or postmenopausal patients were on HRT. Ever since, only a few are. But *all* of them, then and now, told me that they are in a constant battle with their weight. The North American Menopause Society has also confirmed that HRT has no effect on weight gain.

My patients are ecstatic with relief when they realize that their menopause metabolism caused their **MD Factor**. I believe them when they say that they *have* eaten less and exercised more but that nothing worked. And they were even more relieved when I explained why low-calorie plans and restrictive eating simply do not work on the menopause-triggered **MD Factor**, and in some cases can make the problem worse.

When your estrogen levels drop, your metabolism shifts, too—and it needs to be treated differently and fed differently. The problem can't be solved simply by replacing reproductive hormones. But it *can* be solved with the **MD Factor** Action Plan!

Not every hot flash in menopause is caused by unstable blood sugar, but my patients appreciate being able to decrease their episodes by 30 percent or more with something as safe and effective as changing the way they eat. The **MD Factor** Action Plan is designed to stabilize the blood sugar fluctuations that so commonly occur with menopause. And women who lose just 9 percent of their starting body weight have fewer hot flashes compared to women who do not lose any weight.

The More You Gain,
The More You Gain!

Once you start gaining weight, you know how hard it is to get those pounds off. There is a very simple explanation: gaining weight results in changes to your body chemistry. Yes, your metabolism itself actually shifts. You might have thought that nothing's different except your dress size, but ignoring this fact is one of the reasons losing weight is so frustrating.

The body's natural set point for weight differs from person to person, but once you cross the line that's *your* trigger, that fat tissue you now have secretes chemicals that have diabolical effects. Yes, they cause your body to develop even more of the **MD Factor**. Your old metabolism is replaced with a totally different one. And this new metabolism is really, really good at storing fat. That means the old approach to weight loss—taking in fewer calories than you expend—doesn't consistently work anymore.

Most of my overweight patients find that their metabolism shifts noticeably when they're about thirty or more pounds over their normal weight. The **MD Factor** has kicked in so strongly that they can't lose any weight—and in fact often pack on more pounds even when eating the same (or less). What might have once worked for weight loss is now a total failure. And, of course, my patients blame themselves when in fact it's simple physiology making their lives miserable.

As I said earlier in this chapter, the **MD Factor** typically causes weight to accumulate in your abdominal area. This is a double whammy, as the location where fat cells accumulate is crucial to the **MD Factor**. Fat isn't just an inert blob of cells. It's active tissue. And tissues have functions. Fat tissue's function is to secrete hormones and inflammatory chemicals.

The old approach to weight loss—taking in fewer calories than you expend—doesn't consistently work anymore.

Those substances travel throughout the body, telling other cells to damage cell membranes and leading into a deeper **MD Factor** state—and *more* weight gain.

Even thin people can have the **MD Factor**, however. It's true that some people seem to have all the luck—they can eat whatever they want and never gain any weight. The explanation is that the genetic lottery blessed them with fewer fat cells to fill up. However, even they are not entirely off the hook. Their weight gain might not be as obvious, but even very thin people have a small amount of visceral fat cushioning their organs. So while thin people might only gain five to ten pounds, if it's all visceral fat, it puts them at risk for the **MD Factor** as well as for all the medical complications the **MD Factor** causes.

Michelle, for example, had always been thin at 5'4" and 118 pounds, but during menopause she initially gained ten pounds, nearly all of it visceral fat. Although she wasn't close to being overweight at 128 pounds, she slowly continued to gain (and you now know why that happens). She also developed high cholesterol and high blood pressure at levels usually seen in a much heavier person. Yes—she had the **MD Factor**!

How I Diagnose the **MD Factor**

Now that you know why you have the **MD Factor**, this section will tell you what you should discuss with your physician. I suggest you consider doing this before you start the **MD Factor** Action Plan, in order to assess your blood sugar levels, insulin levels, and other parameters of metabolic function. When you have baseline figures, you'll be able to see how they'll respond to the **MD Factor** Action Plan.

1. During my initial consultation with a patient, first I do a physical exam. Most of my patients have fat deposits in their abdomen, which is clearly obvious. One of the diagnostic criteria for the **MD Factor** is a waist

measurement greater than 35 inches for a woman and 40 inches for a man. You can easily take your own waist circumference measurement by locating the top of your hipbone and then placing a tape measure evenly around your bare abdomen where you feel the bone. Make sure that the tape is snug but not pushing tightly into your skin, and measure yourself after breathing out normally. (In other words, sucking in your stomach will give you an inaccurate measurement!)

2. Sometimes I will find a dark coloration of the skin around the neck or in skin creases such as armpits and elbows. This condition, called acanthosis nigricans, is a pigment change, not dirt, and is a visible marker of the **MD Factor**. There might also be many small skin tags around the neck and head area, too.

3. Next, I take a blood pressure reading. Elevated blood pressure (135/85 mm Hg or higher in adults without medication to lower it) is an unwelcome sign. Whether or not your high blood pressure is responding to medication, just having it is a risk factor.

4. Finally, I do specific blood tests on all my patients, children included, for the **MD Factor** when I begin treating them for weight management. (You can see which ones I recommend in Appendix B.) I look for elevations of fasting blood sugar (a level over 100 mg/dL), elevations of the fasting insulin level, and high triglycerides, which are a measure of fat in the blood. I often find mild elevations of liver function tests, suggesting that fat is being deposited in the liver. The cholesterol or lipid panel may also show low HDL or "good" cholesterol. This is usually seen in combination with high triglycerides.

As I mentioned earlier in the section about the **MD Factor** quiz, almost 90 percent of the patients I see in my practice show clear evidence of the **MD Factor** in their blood work, and another 5 percent are very close to testing positive as well on one or more parameters of testing I use. Discuss these tests with your physician or nurse practitioner in order

Do You Have Metabolic Syndrome?

Metabolic syndrome is the advanced form of the **MD Factor**, and a very scary fact is that 30 percent of all American adults—and 47 percent of adults over the age of fifty—have it. You'll need blood work for a firm diagnosis and will need to have at least three of the five findings in this list:

✔ Elevated fasting blood sugar (over 100 mg/dL)

✔ Elevated triglycerides (above 150 mg/dL)

✔ HDL cholesterol level of less than 50 mg/dL for women and less than 40 mg/dL for men

✔ Elevated blood pressure (135/85 mm Hg or higher)

✔ Waist circumference greater than 35 inches for women and greater than 40 inches for men.

to prove if you have the **MD Factor,** and then, most important, follow the values of the MD Factor plan to ensure continual improvement in your weight loss goals. In order for your metabolic dysfunction to be corrected for good, which allows you to keep your weight optimal long term, any abnormal laboratory tests need to normalize.

How My Medical Practice Treats the **MD Factor**

Patients who come to my comprehensive weight management clinic work one-on-one with a clinical nutritionist for at least twelve weeks to develop and modify customized meal plans for weight loss. But that's only the beginning. Everyone needs a long-term plan, and I firmly believe that understanding nutritional basics is extremely important for your continued success. This became clear to me many years ago, when I realized that my patients, so successful in other areas of their lives, had little accurate knowledge about nutrition and more specifically about how their metabolisms responded to food. Very few of the thousands of children, teens, women, and men I've treated had ever heard of the **MD Factor**, much less understood what blood sugar problems were doing to their dieting.

In the remaining chapters in Part II, I'm going to teach you all the basics you need to know about the three main macronutrients—protein, carbohydrates, and fat—that provide most of your calories. You'll also read about an additional source of calories: the alcohol you might be drinking. I'll discuss vitamins, supplements, and exercise, too.

CHAPTER 4

The Protein You Need

Of all the nutrients our bodies need for various functions, protein is the most vital. You need it to build and maintain muscles, tendons, and ligaments; to keep your circulatory system, brain, and all other organs functioning; to keep your immune system healthy and your skin vibrant; and just about everything else! If protein isn't available from food when your body needs it, your tissues start to break down and your organs aren't able to function with optimal power. This can wreak havoc on your cells and your metabolism.

Proteins are made from chains of up to twenty amino acids. Of these twenty, nine are considered to be "essential," because our bodies can't synthesize them. We can only get them by eating protein-rich food. The remaining eleven amino acids can be made in your body from remnants of leftover carbohydrates, fats, and other amino acids.

Foods containing all nine essential amino acids are called complete or high-quality proteins. Those containing less than the essential nine are incomplete or low-quality proteins. Most animal proteins fall into the category of complete or high-quality proteins: meat, poultry, fish, eggs, milk, cheese, and other dairy products. With the exception of soy, proteins from plant sources, vegetables, grains, and fruits are incomplete.

Vegetarians will be the first to tell you that it's not necessary to eat animal protein to have a balanced and healthful diet. But you do have to combine incomplete or low-quality proteins so that you're getting all nine essential amino acids. One of the classic examples is rice and beans. Rice is low in the amino acid lysine and high in the amino acid methionine, whereas beans are low in methionine but high in lysine. They're complementary proteins: served together, they provide a complete protein meal.

One of the challenges for vegetarians who want to lose weight is to take in the essential amino acids needed while limiting excess carbohydrate. Beans and rice are complementary proteins, but the starchy rice is not an ideal food when you have the **MD Factor**. Vegetarians who eat eggs and dairy products, and pescatarians who eat those plus fish, find it easier to regulate their **MD Factor** while getting enough daily protein.

Facts & Myths about Protein

Very few of my patients understand how much protein they do or don't need and how best to consume it. This isn't their fault, of course. I can't tell you how many times I've read articles that get information about protein totally wrong!

One of the easiest assumptions to make is that if a little protein is good, a lot must surely be better. Some people expect protein to create toned muscles, stamina, and athletic prowess. But that's not true at all—eating a hearty serving of red meat every night will not necessarily make you strong.

These are the most important facts about protein:

✔ Your body is in continuous need of protein, but your body can't store it. In fact, the protein you eat at breakfast is pretty much used up by dinnertime. This makes protein a nutrient that is very different from carbohydrates and fat. (Carbohydrates, in the form of glucose, are stored in our liver and muscles, and of course we store fat in our fat tissue.)

✔ Your body can only use a specific amount of protein at any time.

✔ For each meal, you have to hit a certain level of protein to ensure that your body gets the right signals so that it can absorb the amino acids (the building blocks of protein) it needs. The magic number to allow for this absorption is 25–35 grams of dietary protein. This amount also prevents your muscles from being broken down to meet your needs for protein and amino acids when you're trying to lose weight.

✔ For adults, only 4 to 6 ounces of protein are needed at each meal. This is the equivalent of a small chicken breast—not an enormous burger or steak!

✔ If you eat more than 4 to 6 ounces of protein at a time, your body can't use the extra for building and repair. Instead, your body converts it to glucose for energy—or stores it as fat!

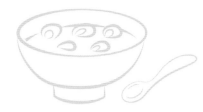

Protein & Dieting

Wouldn't it be wonderful if our bodies only burned the excess fat we are anxious to shed? Unfortunately, nature hasn't been that kind to us!

Not only is the protein we eat broken down to its individual amino acids, but body proteins are constantly being disassembled and reassembled. Muscle proteins, for example, are broken down and quickly re-formed into muscle tissue as well as into other protein-containing tissues such as tendons, blood, and even bone. During this process, called protein turnover, most amino acids are transformed into other amino acids and then used by the tissues in your body. Some, however, are discarded and excreted in your urine. This is why the protein you eat, which replaces these discarded amino acids, is so important in weight loss. If you don't eat enough protein every day, your body will *always* perceive this as a threat to its survival. So it slows down your metabolism, conserving what protein there is, which makes it harder for you to lose weight.

If you eat enough protein, however—in the proper amounts, at regular intervals during the day—this will help keep your metabolism running at an optimal level. And anyone following a low-calorie diet needs *extra* protein to ensure that the body doesn't break down muscle tissue.

How Much Protein Do You Really Need Every Day?

Many people ask me if high-protein diets are bad. The first part of my answer is that you need to understand what "high protein" actually means. Some of my patients find the meal plans I suggest to be higher in protein than they are used to, but that's usually because they've been on protein-*deficient* diets.

When low-fat diets became popular in the 1980s, their proponents insisted that protein and fat were bad for weight loss and that the best way to lose weight was by eating lots of low-calorie carbohydrates. That way of thinking has, unfortunately, persisted—and if you have the **MD Factor**, that's one of the main reasons it's so hard for you to lose weight. When you're not meeting your nutrient requirements each day, your body becomes metabolically hungry and goes into starvation and fat storage mode. At the same time, it sends out intense hunger signals. It's a double whammy: a slower metabolism coupled with cravings for lots of food. The **MD Factor** Action Plan is designed to prevent that from happening.

For about thirty years, the Dietary Guidelines for Americans recommended that we get 15 percent of our calories from protein, 30 percent from fat, and 55 percent from carbohydrate. These percentage-based recommendations make sense for only a small subset of the American population, and they never work for someone who is cutting calories in order to diet.

For example, an active young man eating 3,500 calories a day will take in 130 grams of protein—enough to keep his muscles healthy—if he gets 15 percent of his calories from protein. But if a woman consuming 1,200 calories followed those same recommendations, she'd be getting only

> When you're not meeting your nutrient requirements each day, your body becomes metabolically hungry and goes into starvation and fat storage mode.

45 grams of protein every day. A man on an 1,800-calorie diet would be getting a mere 68 grams of protein. That is just not enough. It means you'll lose muscle tissue as you lose weight. This is unbelievably disconcerting—especially since the RDA (Recommended Daily Allowance) of protein simply to prevent deficiency is 63 grams per day, and that's just a bare minimum. Talk about contradictory advice!

The truth is, most American women ingest an average of 68 grams of protein every day. This is just barely above the amount needed to prevent deficiency, and it's certainly not enough to sustain a regular exercise routine that is meant to strengthen muscles.

Getting back to the question about high-protein diets, it is crucial for you to see why your daily protein requirement is a lot higher than the ridiculously low 15 percent figure put out by the government all those years ago. It is important to note that several years ago, the recommendation changed to ranges: 10–35 percent of calories from protein, 45–65 percent from carbohydrate, and 20–35 percent from fat. This was done because there has been great controversy regarding the proper amount of macronutrients (protein, fat, and carbohydrate) and also because obesity has reached epidemic proportions among the American population in the past thirty years. In addition, research showed that one recommendation was not going to suffice for the entire, extremely varied population.

What is interesting is that the new ranges fit very nicely into what I recommend for my patients in terms of protein amounts. If a woman eats 1,200 to 1,400 calories on a weight loss diet and gets 35 percent of those calories from protein, she is getting 105 to 122 grams of protein. Her carbohydrate intake will be just a little too high at the 45 percent mark and the fat may be just a little low, but those numbers are still pretty close.

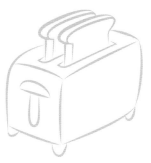

Since the focus of my entire career has been nutrition and metabolism, I was aware of these changes in recommended protein intake, but outside of my medical specialty, this news got very little press. Most people still think that a healthful balanced diet is composed primarily of starchy carbohydrates, because that's what was depicted on the base of the Food Pyramid Guide, a graphic tool formerly used to illustrate how Americans should be eating. What a mistake! I grew up looking at cereal and cracker boxes and bags of chips that had the Food Guide Pyramid graphic on them, showing that for an ideal diet we should be eating six to eleven servings of grains and starches and very little protein and fat. That visual has stayed with most people. No doubt the endless commercials advertising a bowl of cereal with two pieces of toast and a glass of juice as a "complete and balanced breakfast" have also played a lasting role in our perceptions of healthful eating.

Just as you need calcium for strong bones, you need protein for a strong metabolism.

Protein Requirements Designed Specifically for Your Metabolism

I've found that the best way to determine your daily protein requirements is by using *grams* of protein, rather than a percentage of total calories in the diet. Whether you are in the initial weight loss phase or the maintenance phase of the **MD Factor** Action Plan, you will need to eat the same amount of protein. Just as you need calcium for strong bones, you need protein for a strong metabolism.

For patients in my office, I can be very specific with their daily protein recommendations, based on specific parameters such as body composition, a physical exam, and blood work results. For you, the guidelines I'll suggest here are just as helpful, based on calculations that I know are successful for maintaining lean muscle tissue.

I set protein recommendations based on the amount of lean body mass a person has. The lean body mass is the weight of your muscle, organs, bones, and water—everything that's not fat. The lean body mass is what we want to preserve during the process of weight loss. I don't want you to lose bone mass, become dehydrated, or suffer a decline in organ function. The only thing I want you to get rid of is extra body fat.

There will be variations in the amount of lean body mass from one person to another, but not as much as most people think. Women's bones and internal organs are smaller than men's and the size of their muscles is smaller as well. This is why women and men have different recommendations for protein intake.

Your lean body mass should be the same whether you are normal weight or overweight. When we gain weight, we predominantly gain fat tissue, not muscle tissue and organ tissue. It is true that the muscles of overweight people can become larger because they have to carry more weight around on a daily basis. However, the **MD Factor** can cause a loss of muscle tissue and even deposition of fat into muscle fibers as you age.

The bottom line is, with a few exceptions, coming up with the amount of protein your body needs to defeat the **MD Factor**, lose fat, and maintain your muscle tissue is pretty easy. For a woman of average height, which in the United States is 5'4", I recommend 110–120 grams of protein per day. For a man of average height, which in the United States is 5'11", I recommend 130–140 grams of protein per day.

Are there any exceptions?

✔ If a woman or man is between 5' and 5'2", I recommend 100 grams of protein.

✔ If a woman is above 5'10", I recommend 130–140 grams of protein. I would also consider this higher protein intake for a woman who is 5'8" but very muscular.

✔ If a man is taller than 6'2" or is very muscular, he may have a higher protein requirement, 150–160 grams. I don't find we have to go too much higher than this in my practice, but our clientele doesn't include many body builders!

In healthy people, the only known side effect of eating too much protein is what happens if you take in too many calories—you'll gain weight. However, some people have to limit their protein intake due to the fact that their kidneys are not working properly. Protein is a large molecule, and if the kidneys are diseased, the extra work involved in processing it can further strain the kidneys. However, if you have normally functioning kidneys, protein intake does not damage them. For more information, see Appendix A, which discusses in more detail higher protein diets and health concerns.

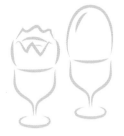

Why Eating Protein at Breakfast Is So Important

One thing nutritionists can agree on is that breakfast is the most important meal of the day.

While you're sleeping, your body is busy breaking down protein to meet its amino acid requirements. If you eat the right amount of protein after this overnight fast, this breakdown stops and, instead, your body primes your metabolism for fat breakdown. But if you don't get enough protein at breakfast, your body will do anything it can to get the protein it needs. That means it'll rob your muscle tissues for it, which is the last thing you want!

Your Protein Needs as You Age

We tend to become less active as we age, and when our energy expenditure goes down, we typically need fewer calories. But our protein needs actually remain *constant*. This is the only way to preserve the lean muscle tissue we have.

In other words, the same man who needed 3,500 calories and 130 grams of protein every day when he's twenty years old and active still needs 130 grams of protein when he's fifty. Unless he's still fantastically fit and active, however, he will not need as many calories. As we all know, though, it can be very hard to alter our eating habits after decades of particular kinds of meals and portion sizes!

What you should do as you age is ensure your consistent intake of protein but cut back on the amount of carbohydrates you eat. You can also slightly decrease your fat intake, but eating fewer carbs will be more effective. You'll see how to do this in the **MD Factor** Action Plan. Increasing your exercise and overall activity levels is also great for your health and general well-being.

Whatever you choose to do, don't cut down on that protein! You need it now more than ever.

In addition, there's leucine, one of the twenty amino acids, to consider, because, as we've seen, it helps regulate the **MD Factor**. When you start the day with adequate leucine levels, you'll have more efficient insulin regulation, which means stabilized blood sugar levels. This also means better weight loss and fewer cravings.

In order to ensure that the right amount of leucine is available when it is most needed first thing in the morning, you must eat close to 25–30 grams of protein at breakfast. This is *essential*. I know it can be tough, as many people just aren't hungry when they get up. They don't like eating breakfast. Plus, a typical breakfast of eggs, bacon, and sausage will meet your protein requirement but is laden with artery-clogging saturated fat.

But what happens if you have a high-carbohydrate meal instead? It triggers the **MD Factor**. Your cells lock out the glucose that is banging on the door to get in. This then trips the signal for more insulin to be released, which later drops blood sugar and sends "I'm starving! Feed me!" signals to your brain. These signals create intense cravings for sugars and carbs during the day. Then you've got a vicious cycle of hunger and cravings in place. Instead of maintaining lean muscle tissue, you'll either break it down or put on fat tissue instead.

My breakfast-resistant patients often balk at first, but they quickly learn that they will lose weight when they eat the right kind of breakfast. It's non-negotiable; it's just a must-do. You *must* start your metabolic engine every morning. And it needs protein to run. These patients are also pretty amazed that once they start eating breakfast regularly, they actually look forward to fueling their bodies properly.

In Chapter 11, I'll provide you with breakfast meal plans that show you exactly what to eat.

One thing nutritionists can agree on is that breakfast is the most important meal of the day.

CHAPTER 5

The Carbohydrates You Need

Picture a twelve-ounce can of Coke. Pour half of it out. What's left in the six ounces of Coke that remains is almost 20 grams of pure sugar.

These 20 grams are equal to all the carbohydrates you should ever get from sugar every day if you want to lose weight, prevent diabetes, and live a long, healthy life.

Shocking, right? But overestimating your body's need for carbs and sugar is as common as underestimating its need for protein. Too many carbs and too little protein mean you will find it nearly impossible to lose weight.

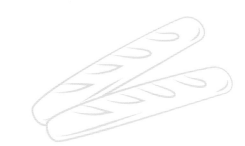

Carbohydrates: You Don't Need as Much as You Think

Carbs are the foundation of most American diets. Believe it or not, carbs are also the foundation of most packaged "diet" foods you can buy in the supermarket. Most Americans get more than half of their calories from carbohydrate sources—primarily sourced from sugar.

Carbohydrates and sugars are practically impossible to avoid. They're in nourishing, sugar-laden breast milk, naturally made tasty and sweet so babies will want to suckle; in your grandmother's famous peach pie and your mom's comforting macaroni and cheese; in the healthful apple you're crunching on and the caramel dipping sauce that makes it taste even better. A heaping bowl of spaghetti and meat sauce is mostly carbs. Make a sandwich of turkey on whole-grain bread and you're still getting more calories from the carbs in the bread than from any other nutrient, such as the protein in the turkey or the fat in the mayonnaise.

Added sugars are also hidden in processed foods you might not think of as sweetened: ketchup, barbecue sauce, baked beans, fat-free salad dressings, granola bars, coleslaw, instant oatmeal, and crackers. These foods taste yummy and are so easy to eat. We are hard-wired to crave and delight in the sweet taste of sugar, and most of us are programmed from an early age to believe that sweets are a treat. You might have been told that if you ate up all your peas and carrots, you'd get a cookie as a reward. Really, who ever heard of getting a stalk of broccoli or a bowlful of raw kale as a treat? Not me!

So what's the big deal about carbs? Why do you need to count them? *Because they become sugar when they enter your bloodstream.* The **MD Factor** is, as you know, set in motion when the excess sugar in your bloodstream can't get into the cells where it's needed. Instead, it's readily stored in your body. This means you'll gain weight or be unable to lose weight.

Simple & Complex Carbohydrates

There are two kinds of carbohydrates: simple and complex.

Simple Carbohydrates

Simple carbohydrates have single or double sugar molecules and are very easy to digest. Glucose and fructose are both simple carbohydrates. They're found in white sugar, high-fructose corn syrup, milk, and fruit juice.

A very common and metabolically dangerous simple sugar is high-fructose corn syrup (or HFCS). HFCS alters hormonal patterns in the body that promote increased body fat and increased appetite. It's mostly metabolized by the liver, and unless you follow up HFCS consumption with exercise, it can get converted into fat stored in and around your liver. In fact, you can get a form of liver disease called non-alcoholic fatty liver disease (NAFLD) just from consuming too much HFCS!

In addition, adults who consume 25 percent of their daily calories as fructose- or HFCS-sweetened beverages (such as soda) for two weeks experience increases in serum levels of cholesterol and triglycerides. The American Heart Association recommends keeping added sugars below 5 percent of your total calories. This is under 25 grams of sugar per day, or about the same amount that is in 8 fluid ounces of soda.

The Most Common Simple Carbohydrates

- Baked goods, including cakes, cookies, doughnuts, pastries, and pies*
- Candy, like chocolate*
- Candy, like jelly beans
- Chips*
- Gum
- Dried fruit
- Fruit juice
- Frozen yogurt, ice cream,* ice pops, sherbet
- Gelatin desserts
- Jelly and jam
- Pretzels
- Processed/refined grains (white flour, white rice)
- Pudding*
- Soft drinks and soda
- Syrups
- Yogurt, sweetened

*Also high in fat

Complex Carbohydrates

Complex carbohydrates consist of long chains of sugar units, which make them taste starchy instead of sweet. Like sugar, complex carbohydrates provide energy. *Unlike* sugars, however, starches are often found in foods rich in vitamins, minerals, and fiber. Because of these nutrients, the body takes a longer time to digest them. This slows down your blood sugar rise and allows your body to utilize them better. In addition, your body is less prone to storing complex carbohydrates as fat, unless they are refined or eaten in large amounts all at one time. It's always better to eat complex rather than simple carbohydrates.

Moreover, eating nothing but a piece of fruit for what you think is a truly healthful snack can cause a larger spike in your blood sugar when you have the **MD Factor**. So what you thought was good for you can actually make you *more* hungry.

And then there's juice. One of the easiest ways to send your blood sugar soaring is by drinking fruit juice, particularly on an empty stomach. Despite the ads you've seen for years, fruit juice is not a healthful food. I never drink it and discourage everyone from even having it in the house, as it's so tempting to drink a lot of it (a normal serving of orange juice is meant to be only 4 ounces—and who drinks that little?). If you are a juice lover, try mixing veggie juices with fruit juice; sweet vegetables like carrots and beets give lots of flavor without so much sugar. Then, gradually try to wean yourself off fruit juices altogether.

When you're in the mood for fruit, portion size matters—a *lot*. Always try to eat fruit with some form of protein (this protein can be a few nuts or a small piece of cheese), as that will slow down its digestion and help moderate any blood sugar spikes.

How Your Body Uses Carbohydrates

As carbohydrates are digested, they are broken down into simple sugars. Your liver then processes them into a form all cells can use—glucose, or blood sugar, which then circulates throughout your body, supplying energy to all tissues and organs that need it.

Glucose has two main destinations after you eat it: it can be absorbed into lean muscle and body cells to be used for energy, or it can be stored as fat. Let me explain. Sometimes your body takes in extra glucose that you don't end up using at that particular time, so the excess is converted

Sugar Hiding in Plain Sight

If you want to spot added sugars on food labels, it can require some detective work. When you investigate the ingredients list, remember that all of the ingredients are listed in descending order by amount. So the food listed first is present in the highest amount, and the ingredient listed last makes up the smallest portion of that food. This list shows you ingredients that indicate added sugar:

- Agave nectar
- Brown sugar
- Barley malt syrup
- Cane crystals
- Cane sugar
- Confectioner's sugar
- Corn sweetener
- Corn syrup
- Corn syrup solids
- Crystalline fructose
- Dehydrated cane juice
- Dextrin
- Dextrose
- Evaporated cane juice
- Fructose
- Fruit juice concentrates
- Glucose
- Glucose syrup
- High-fructose corn syrup
- Granulated sugar
- Honey
- Invert sugar
- Lactose
- Maltodextrin
- Maltose
- Malt syrup
- Maple syrup
- Molasses
- Nectar
- Raw sugar
- Rice syrup
- Saccharose
- Sorghum
- Sorghum syrup
- Sucrose
- Sugar
- Syrup
- Treacle
- Turbinado sugar
- Xylose

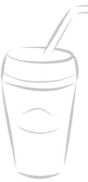

to either glycogen or fat. Glycogen is a starch that is stored in the liver and muscles; it's stashed away in case your body needs it as a quick energy source. Think of it as linking up a bunch of glucose molecules in a row, and then your body breaks off one at a time to use for energy.

But when your glycogen stores are full, the excess glucose takes a different route. It gets converted to *fat*. Unfortunately for all of us, there is no limit to the amount of fat that can be stored by our bodies. And eating excess carbohydrates creates a perfect equation for extra stored fat.

Another important component has to do with carbohydrate tolerance, which is your body's ability to metabolize and use nutrients from the carbs you eat. This is unique to each person and is determined by hepatic regulation (how your liver processes it) and peripheral usage (which refers to how well your cells use energy and respond to blood sugar levels). The factors that affect carbohydrate tolerance are your diet, muscle mass, physical activity, age, and gender.

About High-Fructose Corn Syrup

High-fructose corn syrup (HFCS) is in the news these days, which is a good thing—it helps draw attention to the fact the HFCS is terrible for your body. Unfortunately, however, packaged-food manufacturers still use it because it's inexpensive.

HFCS is bad for you not only because it's sweeter than other forms of sugar but also because it has a different effect on your appetite than other sugars do. HFCS contributes to overeating because it doesn't signal your brain that your stomach is full and you're no longer hungry. Food and drinks that contain regular refined sugar (sucrose) are able to send these signals.

For example, a twenty-two-year-old male athlete will have a high carbohydrate tolerance. He'll have lots of muscle mass due to his youth, his gender (high testosterone levels increase carbohydrate tolerance), and his high level of physical activity. His body processes those carbs as soon as he eats them; his muscles will be sending out signals that they need a lot of fuel so they can exert a lot of energy. This is why so many elite athletes engage in carbohydrate loading before their events—they know that scarfing down bowls of pasta will lead them to peak performance. If you're not an athlete, however, or if you don't work in a profession with high energy needs, such as construction work, you likely won't have high carbohydrate tolerance at all.

It's interesting to note that the recommendations on the old Food Guide Pyramid were unwittingly misleading because they were based on information gathered from active men in the military, for whom a high carbohydrate diet is ideal. But what about a middle-aged office worker who spends most of his time on a computer at his desk? What about women, who on average will have significantly less lean muscle tissue than young men, regardless of activity level? They'll look to the Dietary Guidelines for Americans or the outdated Food Guide Pyramid for guidance and end up eating in a way that will pack the pounds right on. They need the **MD Factor** Action Plan to undo the damage!

The Most Common Complex Carbohydrates

VEGETABLES

The best choice of carbohydrates will always be vegetables. These all have very low carbohydrate content and are rich in fiber and nutrients.

- Artichokes
- Arugula
- Asparagus
- Bean sprouts
- Beets
- Broccoli
- Brussels sprouts
- Cabbage
- Carrots
- Cauliflower
- Celery
- Cucumbers
- Eggplants
- Green beans
- Greens (collard, mustard, turnip)
- Kale
- Leeks
- Lettuce
- Mushrooms
- Okra
- Onions
- Peppers (all colors)
- Radishes
- Sauerkraut
- Spinach
- Shallots
- Snow peas
- Spaghetti squash
- Squash (summer or winter)
- Tomatoes
- Wax beans
- Zucchini

BEANS AND LEGUMES

The next best carbohydrates are beans and legumes. Chock full of amino acids, they're particularly rich in fiber, which helps you feel full.

- Black beans
- Black-eyed peas
- Chickpeas
- Green peas
- Kidney beans
- Lentils
- Navy beans
- Red beans
- White beans

FRUITS

Fruit is rich in phytonutrients, fiber, and the sweet sugar fructose. (See the sidebar on the right for more about how much fruit to eat.) Because fruit has a high sugar content, you don't want to eat it in unlimited quantities.

- Apples
- Applesauce, unsweetened
- Apricots
- Bananas
- Blackberries
- Blueberries
- Boysenberries
- Cantaloupe
- Cherries
- Clementines
- Cranberries
- Dates
- Grapefruit
- Grapes
- Honeydew
- Kiwis
- Mandarin oranges
- Mangos
- Nectarines
- Oranges
- Papayas
- Peaches
- Pears
- Persimmons
- Pineapple
- Plums
- Strawberries
- Raspberries
- Tangerines
- Watermelon

WHOLE GRAINS AND STARCHY VEGETABLES

Grains tend to have a higher carbohydrate count than other carbs, especially due to the enormous portions that are often considered to be a single serving. Most people with the **MD Factor** need to pay careful attention to their grain intake and eat appropriately sized portions of fiber-rich grains such as steel-cut oatmeal or whole-wheat bread. You'll see exactly what's best for you on the **MD Factor** Action Plan in Chapter 11.

- Barley
- Brown rice
- Corn
- Oats
- Potatoes
- Quinoa
- Rye
- Wheat

Watch Your Fruit Consumption!

"Eat your fruit and vegetables!" How many times did you hear that growing up?

Fruit is an amazing food, loaded with vitamins, minerals, fiber, and phytonutrients that are great for your body. But here's the thing you need to know: most fruits are laden with simple sugars that are easy to digest. You can eat a lot of fruit before it makes you feel full—and that means you are eating a lot of sugar that can trigger your **MD Factor**.

Carbohydrates are not a
dieter's enemy—all vegetables
contain carbs, and so do
all fruits.

Facts & Myths about Carbohydrates

My patients often come to see me with a lot of misinformation about how much and what kind of carbohydrates to eat. It's important to emphasize that carbohydrates are not a dieter's enemy—all vegetables contain carbs, and so do all fruits. It's eating the *wrong kind* of carbs at the wrong time that causes weight problems. The right type of carbohydrates, such as those found in vegetables, legumes, and low-sugar fruits, form the backbone of good nutrition.

Nutritionally, there is no such thing as an essential carbohydrate. Carbs are not needed for our survival. It's hard to believe, I know. (You should see my patients' faces when I tell them this!) But as long as the human body has stored fat and adequate muscle mass, we can live without carbs. However, we cannot live without protein and fat, as our bodies need specific amino acids from protein and fatty acids from fat that we cannot manufacture. Without carbs, on the other hand, your body makes glucose from protein and ketones from fat for the fuel it needs. For example, the Inuit peoples, native to Alaska and other northern areas, ate a high-protein, high-fat diet (an average of 75 percent of calories from fat) essentially devoid of dietary carbohydrates. They consume lots of fatty fish like salmon and halibut and hunt for walrus, whales, caribou, and seal, and are able to thrive.

Another thing you may find hard to believe is that sugar is not the best thing to eat when your blood sugar drops. When you have the **MD Factor**, eating simple carbs is absolutely the worst thing to do! Not only will it act like an appetite stimulant, but any excess sugar that you eat will be stored as fat. And then you'll likely be even hungrier an hour after eating—hungrier, in fact, than if you'd eaten nothing at all. As you'll see in the **MD Factor** Action Plan, keeping your blood sugar levels steady will prevent these intense hunger pangs, and eating snacks that are rich in other nutrients besides simple carbs will keep the **MD Factor** at bay.

A last myth you may have encountered involves weight loss plateaus. Don't allow plateaus to make you give up! If you've tried a low-carbohydrate diet before, you might have lost weight for several weeks or months and then hit a frustrating plateau. Don't despair. In Appendix A, "Why Other Diets Don't Work," I'll tell you why these diets failed for you—and why the **MD Factor** Action Plan *will* work.

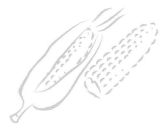

How Many Carbohydrates Do You Really Need Every Day?

When you have the **MD Factor**, the best sources of carbohydrates are vegetables, legumes, and low-sugar fruit. The next best sources are complex starches such as sweet potatoes or whole-grain bread. You'll need to keep an eye on how many grams of carbohydrates you're taking in. Intake is measured in grams, and food labels will list how many grams of carbohydrates and sugar are in each serving of food. Be sure to check the size of each serving, as eating too large a serving is an all-too-easy way of going over your carb target. In Appendix F, you'll see a helpful list of the best carbs to eat, with a breakdown of their protein, carb, fat, and fiber contents.

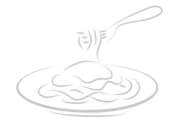

How to Calculate Your Daily Carbohydrate Intake

To correct the **MD Factor**, keep your total carb intake to between 60 and 100 grams, spread throughout the day. This will keep insulin release to a minimum, maintain a stable blood sugar level, and stop those hunger pangs before they happen. It will also improve your energy level and ensure that these carbs don't get stored as fat.

Anytime you eat an apple, a bagel, a bowl of pasta, a piece of white bread, or a candy bar, your blood sugar or glucose level will go up. For example, a normal blood sugar level before eating is 80 mg/dL. For every 15 grams of carbohydrate that gets absorbed into your digestive tract, your blood sugar will rise 30 points. An apple contains about 17 grams of carbohydrates, so when you eat it, your blood sugar will go up to 112 mg/dL. But since the apple's carb content is under the magic number of 20 grams, no insulin is needed to lower your blood sugar, which will soon return to normal as the carbohydrates are metabolized.

Eating or drinking simple carbs on their own, on the other hand—like a bowl of white rice or a large glass of orange juice—will cause blood sugar to rise dramatically, triggering a large insulin spike. If you eat the appropriate portions of high-fiber complex carbohydrates instead, their longer digestion time won't trigger as large a spike in insulin. Even high-fiber complex carbohydrates trigger insulin release if you eat a portion that's too large.

Foods high in lean protein—such as light cheese, low-sugar yogurt, and nuts—do not trigger insulin release. In addition, meals combining protein and carbohydrates cause less of an insulin spike than meals that are solely carb-based. Eating a plain white bagel with a bit of jam is not a good combo; eating half a whole-grain bagel with a few slices of turkey and a slice of low-fat cheese is a much better idea!

Let's Get Real about Carbohydrate Portions

Did you know that a single serving of carbohydrate is one 3-inch square of sliced bread? What kind of sandwich can you make with that? A very tiny one! But at your favorite fast-food chain, a 6-inch sandwich contains the equivalent of three servings of bread—and you haven't put anything on it yet. Grab the foot-long, and you'll be eating *six* servings. That's all the carbohydrates you need for the entire day.

Or what about ordering a delicious bowl of spaghetti Bolognese at your favorite Italian restaurant? A normal serving of pasta is ½ cup of dry pasta, cooked. The serving size you're likely to get, on the other hand, will likely be closer to *4 cups* of pasta, plus the sauce and toppings.

Yes, that's right. An entrée size of spaghetti Bolognese is the equivalent of *eight servings*! Even if you only eat half and take the rest home for another meal, you still will have eaten four servings at once. Add in the restaurant bread, a few bites of your daughter's cheesecake, and a glass or two of wine, and you've ingested enough carbs to last you for days!

Restaurants are a particular problem when it comes to serving sizes. Even the plates, glassware, and utensils have grown. Appetizer plates are the same size that dinner plates used to be, and dinner plates are practically platters. And restaurants that don't supersize their servings to keep up with their competition are restaurants that soon go out of business. But everywhere food is sold—grocery stores, bakeries, delis, specialty stores, and especially fast-food chains—portions are ballooning. The one-size-only 7-Eleven soda grew into a Big Gulp and then a Super Big Gulp. Remember when a muffin was roughly the size of a cupcake, or a bagel was a scant 3 ounces? Not anymore! The muffin contains enough calories, fat, and carbs for two entire meals, and the bagel can practically

What can you do to retrain your brain to accept a smaller size portion of food as the new normal?

be used as a paperweight. Yet researchers find we're still eating the whole thing, without comprehending the alarming increase in our daily caloric intake.

But perhaps the most important consequence of all this commercial supersizing is what it's done to our perception of appropriate portions. As we get used to seeing those big portions when we eat out, we tend to re-create them in our home kitchens, so that even when we do our own cooking, we again serve ourselves more than we need. We've become a supersized nation, and we eat *way* more carbs than we think. My patients are often shocked to see their carbohydrate intake once they start to monitor and record it.

Supersize portions wouldn't be such an issue if we were better at walking away. An old adage about fitness says that the most important exercise to do is "push backs"—as in push back from the table when you've had enough. But many Americans were raised to feel guilty if we left food on our plates. Add that programming to a giant dish of pasta, and suddenly you're stuffed!

The truth is, no matter how we were raised or whether we're slim or overweight, if more food is put in front of us, we'll eat more, period. Usually we're not even aware of this fact—but researchers have proven it in countless studies. During one test, people who unknowingly ate from soup bowls that were surreptitiously being refilled from under the table ate 73 percent more soup than those who were given one normal serving. "How can I be full?" the testers wondered. "I have half a bowl of soup left!" We judge how much we have eaten or how full we are by the amount of food that's left on our plate or in the serving container. We will eat much more out of a larger box or bag or plate.

As the key to carbs and weight loss is to shrink your portions, what can you do to retrain your brain to accept a smaller size portion of food as the new normal?

When You're at Home

- Use smaller plates.

- Serve beverage with calories, such as juice or milk, out of a tall thin glass. We perceive liquids in this shape of vessel as larger than they really are.

- Serve beverages without any calories, such as water or unsweetened iced tea, out of a short, stout glass. We perceive liquids in this shape of vessel as less than they really are. So many people find it hard to get all the water they need—this trick can help you drink the 64 ounces (at least) of water you need every day.

- Use smaller glasses, cups, and serving utensils, too. Swap that dinner fork for a salad fork, and use a slender iced teaspoon instead of a teaspoon or tablespoon.

- Fill the plates from the stove and bring them to the table. Repeated studies have shown that if the food is within arm's reach, we'll eat it. But if we've got to get up for seconds, we're less likely to do so.

- Eat slowly and chew your food well. There's a lag between when your stomach is full and when your brain receives the signal that you're full. If you eat more slowly, you give your brain a chance to catch up with your stomach.

- Don't allow use of electronic devices during family dinners. This means you'll have to talk to each other—and it's really hard to eat a lot when you're engrossed in conversation. Plus, it sets a great example for your family members.

When You're Eating Out

- Order two appetizers instead of an appetizer and an entrée.

- Use a salad fork instead of a dinner fork.

- Ask for the bread basket to be taken away. It's too easy to overeat bread if it's just sitting there.

- Eat half of what's on your plate, and ask your server to pack the rest up for you to take home.

- Eat slowly and chew your food well.

- Drink a lot of water. It helps fill you up.

Your Carbohydrate Needs as You Age

Most people become less active with age, and their muscle mass declines along with their energy levels. These changes are most noticeable in those who are sedentary. Even very fit and active seniors will inevitably lose some muscle mass due to age and declining growth hormone levels—but those losses are much lower than those seen in the sedentary population.

Less muscle mass means there is simply less tissue that needs glucose. That's why the older you get, the less you need to eat. So downsize those portions.

CHAPTER 6

The Fat You Need

Fat is not your enemy! Fats provide support for your cardiovascular, reproductive, immune, and nervous systems. Not only is fat an important nutrient in your diet—it's essential. Severely restricting fat could be life threatening.

In my two decades of working with weight loss, I've learned that the misperceptions about fat are even more stunning than the misperceptions about sugar. Part of the reason for this is that even scientists and nutritionists have gotten it wrong. Back in the 1980s and 1990s, low-fat and non-fat foods were all the rage. Cookies, doughnuts, and candies were reformulated to become fat free and marketed as practically bursting with healthful goodness. Foods that contained healthful fats, such as nuts or avocados, were written off as diet-busters. I look back at this madness and shake my head, because what was the fat in all those foods replaced with? *Sugar*. And what does eating all that sugar do to you? It triggers the **MD Factor**, of course!

Facts & Myths about Fat

Certain types of fat are ones that our bodies can't manufacture. These are the essential fatty acids (EFAs), and we need to eat them in our food. EFAs are used by your body to create every other type of fat you need.

There are two types of EFAs: eicosapentaenoic acid (EPA) and docosahexaenoic acid (DHA). This is what EFAs do:

- They are crucial for proper growth in children, particularly for nerve development and the development of sensory systems.

- They allow your brain to function. Your brain is actually 60 percent fat, primarily DHA. Without fat, you literally can't think!

- They help increase circulation and reduce blood pressure.

- EFAs not only slow the production of cholesterol but also improve the delicate ratio of HDL to LDL cholesterol, as well as reducing the "stickiness" of platelets in your bloodstream, which is essential to reducing the risk of heart disease and stroke. Thinking that all fats will give you high cholesterol levels is one of the biggest fat myths out there!

- EFAs act as a carrier of vitamins in your bloodstream. Without it, the critically important vitamins A, D, E, and K can't be transported properly.

- Good fats protect cells against invading toxins, bacteria, viruses, and allergens, which may help reduce allergies and inhibit the growth of malignant cancer cells.

- EFAs have an important role in your body's biochemistry. You need them to produce prostaglandins, hormone-like substances that control every cell of your body on a second-by-second basis. Consequently, they're essential to body functions such as heart rate, blood pressure, blood clotting, fertility, energy production, oxygen consumption, and maintaining a proper metabolic rate.

- They elevate energy levels, creating stamina and decreasing recovery time from fatigue.

- EFAs also play a huge role in immune function, the process by which your body regulates inflammation and fights infection.

- EFAs form a structural part of all cell membranes. This means they help regulate the traffic of substances into and out of your cells, ensuring that cells can obtain optimal levels of nutrients and expel harmful waste products. This also plays a role in the **MD Factor,** as cell membranes are where your insulin receptors are located. It's vitally important to have healthy cell membranes in order to help reverse insulin resistance.

Why Do We Have Body Fat?

One of the most important roles of body fat is insulation and protection. Body fat insulates us from cold temperatures. Internally, fat provides a cushion for our vital organs, protecting them from trauma and keeping them from being jolted around. This is why even those who appear slender usually have at least 10 percent body fat.

Another major role of body fat is the storage of energy from food for later use. A small amount is stored as carbohydrates (in the form of glycogen) in our liver and muscles, but the most significant source of stored energy is body fat.

Body fat is perfectly designed for the job. It is compact, containing twice the energy of an equal amount of glycogen. And it doesn't need water for storage, as glycogen does. But because our bodies are so remarkably efficient at storing fat, when you have the **MD Factor,** it's all too easy to store fat.

Why Is Enough Dietary Fat Helpful in Metabolism Correction?

Surprisingly enough, fat can also help you control your hunger. Fat takes a long time to digest, so we feel full longer. Fat does not require the release of insulin for digestion and does not trigger blood sugar swings unless the food containing fat also contains sugar. And fat often makes food taste better, which is why some dieters have a tough time cutting down on the amount of fat they eat. They can't imagine a sandwich without mayo, corn on the cob without butter, a salad without a creamy dressing . . . or dessert without whipped cream on top!

Surprisingly enough, fat can also help you control your hunger. Fat takes a long time to digest, so we feel full longer.

Some of the best sources of essential fatty acids are cold-water fish such as salmon, sardines, halibut, cod, tuna, striped bass, and herring. They are also found in oils of plant origin: walnut oil, flaxseed oil, olive oil, mango kernel oil, soybean oil, wheat germ oil, and canola oil.

Good Fat vs. Bad Fat, or Unsaturated vs. Saturated

Not all fats are equal. Let's see why.

All fats are either saturated or unsaturated. The difference between them lies in their chemical structure, particularly the fatty acid chain of each molecule. This chain is made up of oxygen, carbon, and hydrogen atoms. When the spaces for hydrogen atoms are filled to capacity—like the spaces for cars in a parking garage—the fatty acid is saturated. Unsaturated fats have a few parking spaces open, and this makes them more usable by your body.

Saturated Fat

You can always tell a saturated fat, as it's solid at room temperature. Saturated fats should be on your need-to-limit list. The qualities that make them saturated are the qualities that allow them to be deposited in our arteries, leading to diseases of the heart and blood vessels. They also tend to raise cholesterol levels in our blood.

Meats and dairy products provide good-quality protein—but they also are responsible for the majority of saturated fat in the typical American diet. The protein choices listed in the **MD Factor** Action Plan are high in protein but also low in saturated fat.

Foods High in Saturated Fats

- Bacon
- Beef
- Butter
- Cheese
- Cream
- Cream cheese
- Egg yolks
- Half and half
- Lamb
- Lard
- Milk (whole)
- Pork
- Sour cream
- Veal

Two vegetable oils, palm oil and coconut oil, are highly saturated, but as they come from plants, they don't have the same drawbacks as animal-based saturated fats. They're medium-chain fatty acids, with a chemical structure that helps them maintain the integrity of your gastrointestinal tract's lining.

Unsaturated Fat

You can always tell an unsaturated fat, as it's liquid at room temperature. It is much more heart-healthy than saturated fat; some, such as olive oil, may even bring down blood cholesterol levels.

In general, fats from vegetable sources, such as corn oil, cottonseed oil, soybean oil, safflower oil, and sesame oil, are less saturated than those from animals. But watch out—they are often found in processed or junk foods.

Unsaturated fats can be either *mono*unsaturated (missing two hydrogen atoms) or *poly*unsaturated (missing more than two hydrogen atoms). Each affects your blood cholesterol differently. Monounsaturated fats are beneficial because they lower total blood cholesterol levels while increasing the "good" HDL cholesterol. And while some polyunsaturated fats contain beneficial EFAs and also reduce total cholesterol levels, some may have the additional unwanted effect of reducing "good" HDL cholesterol levels, too.

For optimal health, get your vital EFAs from a mix of polyunsaturated and monounsaturated fats. These are the healthful oils made from nuts, seeds, and wild-caught cold-water fish. Be sure to look for minimally processed oils, such as cold-pressed oils.

Polyunsaturated Fats

- Almonds
- Corn oil
- Cottonseed oil
- Flaxseed
- Safflower oil
- Sesame seeds
- Soybeans, soybean oil
- Sunflower seeds, sunflower seed oil
- Walnuts, walnut oil

Monounsaturated Fats

- Almonds
- Avocado
- Canola oil
- Cashews
- Olive oil
- Peanuts, natural peanut butter, peanut oil
- Pecans

Unsaturated Fats Gone Bad: Trans Fats

Unsaturated fats become very unhealthful when they are converted into trans fatty acids, or trans fats. Although a small amount of trans fats are found naturally in foods such as meat, butter, and milk, most trans fat is formed when hydrogen is added to an oil to make it more solid—as is done in the manufacturing of shortening or margarine. This process, called hydrogenation, increases shelf life of these fats, which helps maintain the flavor and texture of processed foods.

The chemical composition of hydrogenated trans fats provides a way of chemically providing the missing hydrogen atoms I mentioned earlier. But they're added in a way that has negative effects on the body's cells. As a result, trans fats are linked to many negative and potentially serious health conditions, including a higher risk for developing diabetes. Eating lots of partially hydrogenated vegetable fat can trigger the **MD Factor**. Trans fats also seem to suppress the levels of "good" HDL cholesterol, and they can elevate triglyceride blood levels as well. These are all markers for a higher risk of heart disease.

Labels indicating the amount of trans fats in packaged foods became mandatory in 2006. According to FDA regulations, "If the serving contains less than 0.5 gram [of trans fat], the content shall be expressed as zero." Talk about tricky packaging! Manufacturers get around this by making the serving sizes small. If a food has 0.4 grams per serving and you eat four servings—not hard to do with junk food like potato chips, where a serving is only eight or nine chips (and who eats so few?), or microwave popcorn—you've just unwittingly consumed 1.6 grams of trans fat, even though the package says there are zero grams of trans fat per serving!

So if the label says zero trans fats, don't believe it. If you see "hydrogenated oil," "partially hydrogenated oil," or "shortening" in the ingredients list, those are trans fats and you've been duped! Your only recourse is to read labels carefully.

You can't do that when you eat out, of course. When you cook at home, you are in complete control of the kind of fat you use, but unless you're in a restaurant's kitchen while they're making your food, there's no way to be sure you are getting food prepared with healthful olive oil instead of unhealthful margarine or shortening. The most common source of dangerous trans fats is fried food. A small order of french fries can deliver anywhere from 4 to 7 grams of trans fat straight to your arteries. Even if these restaurants use liquid oil for frying, the potatoes are often pre-fried in hydrogenated fats before shipping.

The FDA and the Surgeon General recommend that you eliminate all trans fats from your diet, and I agree. Many food manufacturers have replaced trans fats with saturated fats, but that's still an extremely unhealthful choice with little nutritional improvement. Too much fat adds too many calories to your day, and too much trans fat adds all sorts of potential health problems to your body.

Food Sources of Trans Fats

- Baked goods, packaged (cakes, cookies, crackers, muffins, pie crusts)
- Bread (hamburger and hot dog buns)
- Breakfast cereals, sweetened
- Candy bars
- Chips (potato, corn, tortilla)
- Dough, packaged (bake-it-yourself rolls, pizza dough)
- Fried foods (doughnuts, french fries, fried chicken including chicken nuggets, hard taco shells)
- Frosting, canned
- Margarine (stick and some tubs)
- Mayonnaise
- Pasta with sauce, packaged (macaroni and cheese, rice dishes, side dishes, canned pasta)
- Popcorn, microwave
- Pre-mixed baking products (cake mix, pancake mix)
- Pre-mixed drink mixes (hot chocolate, flavored drink mixes added to milk)
- Vegetable shortening

Your Fat Needs as You Age

You still need to ensure you are meeting your essential requirements for fat as you grow older. However, as you age, you also need to ensure that you are not eating more calories than your current activity level allows. If you are eating the protein you need, you will take in fat, as protein foods from both animal and plant sources (meat, fish, nuts) contain fat. Research shows that it is healthier—and reduces the **MD Factor**—to replace carbohydrate calories with calories from healthful fats and protein.

How Much Fat Can You Have While on the **MD Factor** Action Plan?

Just as sugar is hidden in food, so is a lot of fat. You can't see the fat in a glass of milk, in a piece of cheese, or in a brownie. You can see fat in meat (if it is possible to trim it off your steak or roast, please do so), although it's harder to notice in ground beef. This can make it a bit tricky to know how much fat you're really eating. Ideally, you want to eat the right amount to give your body what it needs to function, but not too much so that it increases your weight.

Each gram of fat contains nine calories, whereas protein and carbohydrate only contain four calories. Since fat calories are so concentrated, they can very quickly add up. Nuts, for example, contain protein and healthful fats, but usually twice as much fat as protein. And it's incredibly easy to overeat them when you're trying to lose weight.

Women should take in no more than 30–40 grams of fat per day. (This is about 25–30 percent of the calories on a 1,200-calorie diet.) Men should consume 40–60 grams per day.

It's always best to eat foods containing EFAs and monounsaturated fats. Limit your consumption of saturated fats, and stay far away from trans fats as much as possible.

The easiest way to limit the amount of fat you eat is by primarily eating real foods and avoiding processed foods. If you do need to rely on processed, packaged foods for convenience reasons, you have to become an expert label reader. Look at the Nutrition Facts label and read the ingredients list. Keep in mind that the front of the box or package can be deliberately misleading as a marketing ploy.

Remember, you need to eat the right amount of protein, but to lose weight, calories still matter. And higher-fat foods have more calories.

CHAPTER 7

The Vitamins and Supplements You Need

Some nutrients are more important than others when it comes to weight loss and correcting your **MD Factor**. I specifically test magnesium levels, vitamin D levels, and vitamin B12 levels in my patients who have the **MD Factor**. These three nutrients are extremely powerful in their ability to fix your metabolism, making them the most relevant to weight loss. They help you regulate your blood sugar and improve your **MD Factor** in various ways.

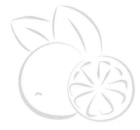

Why We Need Supplements

A vitamin is a small, complex compound that allows certain chemical reactions in the body to take place. We need them to extract energy from foods and to build and repair our bodies, as well as to keep our cells healthy and protected.

When I was in medical school, we were taught that if we ate a healthful diet, we wouldn't need to take any vitamins or supplements. And in an ideal world, all of our nutrients would be provided to us in the food we eat. But that rarely happens, and you can still be surprisingly deficient even if you have an excellent diet. There are several reasons:

- Modern industrial farming practices often don't transfer important minerals back into the soil, so the produce from that soil can be deficient in minerals.

- The tomato you buy in Boston may have been picked in California up to a week or two earlier, and fruit that doesn't fully ripen on the vine contains far fewer nutrients than fruit that is picked ripe just before you consume it.

- Certain medical conditions and/or medications affect absorption. Many people take acid-blocking medications to help decrease stomach acid and heartburn symptoms. These medications affect the absorption of important nutrients, such as vitamin B12 and magnesium. In addition, Metformin, used for the treatment of the **MD Factor** as well as diabetes, can also impair the absorption of vitamin B12. (For more about metformin, see Appendix E.)

- High stress levels increase the excretion of nutrients.

- Intense athletic training can deplete nutrients.

- And then there's dieting!

The truth is, it's hard to get all the vitamins and minerals you need from your food alone, so it's a good idea to take a basic, high-potency multivitamin-mineral supplement daily.

Furthermore, I've learned during my years in practice that for those who are constantly dieting, vitamin levels can fluctuate—a lot! This has convinced me that many people need *more* than just a daily multivitamin.

The trouble is, there is so much conflicting information in the media about supplementation that my patients are very confused about what's best for them. You practically need a nutrition degree to decipher it all!

You can still be surprisingly deficient even if you have an excellent diet.

The Best Daily Supplements for Weight Loss

Adding quality nutrients, especially if you have one or more deficiencies, will help supercharge your **MD Factor** Action Plan. Not only will they work synergistically to lessen the **MD Factor**'s effects on your cells, but they also promote a healthy detoxification of your liver, which is essential for successful weight loss. This list contains everything that I recommend for most of my patients.

Vitamins and Minerals

- Vitamin D3
- Vitamin B12
- Magnesium
- Chromium
- Folic acid (as methylfolate)

Other Supplements

- Alpha lipoic acid
- Cinnamon
- ECGC (from green tea)
- N-acetylcysteine
- Omega-3 oil (from fish oil)

Herbal Supplements

- Berberine

You would be amazed at how many Americans are severely deficient in Vitamin D.

Vitamin D Can Reduce the **MD Factor**

You would be amazed at how many Americans are severely deficient in vitamin D. My office is located in Naples, Florida, yet even local patients who are exposed to sunshine year-round are seriously lacking in this vitamin, much to their shock!

Vitamin D allows calcium to be absorbed and placed into your bones. It also is responsible for proper mood state, because it influences how certain neurotransmitters, such as serotonin, are produced. Most cells in your body have receptors for vitamin D, and there is an overwhelming amount of research related to vitamin D's ability to reduce inflammation and to increase immune response.

But most important for my **MD Factor** patients, vitamin D can improve your sensitivity to insulin. Countless studies have shown that this one vitamin has major benefits when it comes to the **MD Factor**. People with higher blood levels of vitamin D are less likely to have diabetes. Other studies have shown that increasing vitamin D levels from a low range to a normal range greatly improves insulin sensitivity by up to 60 percent. Improving insulin sensitivity is exactly what this book is all about. When you do that, you defeat the **MD Factor**.

Without enough vitamin D, you can have serious health issues, as this deficiency can lead to any or all of the following:

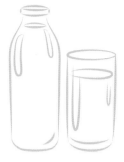

- Autoimmune diseases
- Breast cancer
- Chronic pain
- Colon cancer
- Coronary artery disease
- Depression
- Diabetes

- Gum disease
- Heart attack
- Hypertension (high blood pressure)
- Osteoarthritis
- Osteoporosis
- Prostate cancer
- Stroke

Correcting a vitamin D deficiency is vitally important if you have the **MD Factor**.

VITAMIN D For most adults, the recommended dose of vitamin D is a highly contentious issue. While we know how harmful a vitamin D deficiency is, doctors and nutritionists are not sure what an ideal level should be. You should discuss your options with your physician. I think it's best to take around 2,000 IU per day, and make sure it's D3, not D2. Your body should be able to get what it needs, and you won't be taking enough to have any type of overdose. (Note that you can't overdose on vitamin D through sun exposure, as after your body has made what it needs, additional sun exposure breaks down any excess of the vitamin.) If you're taking a supplement, it's a really good idea to get your vitamin D level checked, to ensure that your level is not too high, which can affect your blood calcium levels.

Reasons for Vitamin D Deficiencies

One of the primary reasons for vitamin D deficiency is related to its ability to dissolve in fat. Because this vitamin is stored in fat tissue, the more weight people gain, the more their fat holds on to vitamin D, leaving less available for use in the bloodstream. This is especially pertinent for anyone who is seriously overweight (meaning their body fat is 30 percent above a normal weight for their height) and who does little outside activity exposing them to the sun.

Sunscreen can also reduce your body's production of vitamin D. While it's important to protect the skin from the sun's two types of ultraviolet rays, UVA (which can cause skin damage and photoaging) and UVB (which causes sunburn and skin cancer), UVB is needed to produce vitamin D. Light-skinned individuals need only fifteen to twenty minutes of exposure to the sun each day (and only a portion of the skin needs to be exposed, too, not the whole body) to synthesize adequate amounts of vitamin D, about the equivalent of 10,000 IU. For those of us who have darker skin, we need about an hour of exposure. And the skin of older people can synthesize only 25 percent as much vitamin D as the skin of someone decades younger.

Other factors that may contribute to vitamin D deficiencies include diet (if you are lactose intolerant or a vegan, you will normally eat fewer foods fortified with vitamin D, such as dairy products) and malabsorption illnesses (if you have Crohn's disease or cystic fibrosis, you will be at a greater risk of deficiency).

Vitamin D2 or Vitamin D3?

There are two forms of vitamin D available in supplements: D2 and D3. D2 is the inactive, inefficient form, synthesized from plants, and is most commonly used in prescriptions for vitamin D as well as in foods that can then claim to be "fortified with vitamin D." Vitamin D3 is the active form and typically is sourced from animal foods such as cold-water fish or eggs; this is the form your body can more easily use.

I often use much higher doses of pharmaceutical-grade vitamin D3 to correct deficiencies—never D2, as I've found that it doesn't bring levels back up. If you are prescribed a high dose, your blood levels must be monitored to ensure your level is optimal and not too high. Ask your physician to do a 25-OH vitamin D test, and discuss your options.

Vitamin B12 Will Increase Your Energy & Your Metabolism

Vitamin B12 is required for energy production; without enough, your metabolism can plummet. This explains why adequate vitamin B12 levels are crucial when you're trying to lose weight. But because many medications impair its absorption—this includes acid blockers such as Prilosec, Prevacid, and other proton pump inhibitors, as well as metformin, which is used to treat diabetes, pre-diabetes, and the **MD Factor**—vitamin B12 deficiency is something I frequently diagnose in my practice. It's especially prevalent in vegans, as they aren't eating any animal sources of B12. Just getting older also affects the absorption of B12. Symptoms include fatigue, depression, a sore tongue and lips, and numbness and tingling in the hands and feet.

Sometimes a vitamin pill with a higher dosage of B12 is all that's needed to fix the deficiency, but that won't work if your body has trouble absorbing the vitamin. If so, a sublingual tablet or drops gets the B12 vitamin directly into circulation via the blood vessels beneath your tongue. If this is still not enough, 1,000 mcg of B12 can be injected monthly.

I always check the B12 level of all of my patients who are struggling with weight issues and monitor these levels over time to ensure they return to normal. Ask your doctor to check your own levels, especially if you have any of the symptoms mentioned.

VITAMIN B12 The dose of vitamin B12 suggested by the FDA is 6 mcg daily. It's best for adults over the age of fifty to obtain most of their vitamin B12 from vitamin supplements or fortified foods. However, I recommend 500 mcg per day to my patients, if not more. The sublingual tablets are usually 1,000 mcg and injections are 1,000 mcg monthly. B12 is a safe supplement to take, and it is water soluble, so it does not build up in your system the same way a fat-soluble vitamin such as vitamin D can. However, I would recommend caution with taking these higher doses of B12 if you have kidney disease. (If you have kidney disease, any supplement you take must be approved by your personal physician.)

Magnesium

Magnesium is needed to ensure the efficiency of more than three hundred enzymatic processes in your body. It's necessary for proper blood flow, electrolyte balance, contracting and relaxing muscles, and proper glucose metabolism. For those with the **MD Factor**, it can help correct blood sugar regulation.

Many foods today contain less magnesium than they did fifty years ago because of the changes in farming methodologies. As a result, many of my patients are deficient, especially those with poorly controlled diabetes. This is especially true for those who have chronic constipation, muscle tightness or spasms, high blood pressure, and environmental allergies.

Magnesium comes in many forms, and it's important to take the right kind. Many tablet multivitamins contain magnesium oxide, which is not very well absorbed. In addition, taking too much magnesium by mouth can cause diarrhea; magnesium citrate is the most likely culprit, which is why it's often used as a laxative. Magnesium glycinate or magnesium taurate are a bit gentler on your system.

Keep Your Liver Healthy

We are continuously exposed to fat-soluble chemicals, preservatives, and pesticides—often without our knowledge. Whatever the source, your body treats them as toxins, and as a result they're typically stored in your fat tissues so your vital organs are protected from their effects. But when you lose weight and metabolize fat tissue, those toxins are released into your bloodstream.

Your liver is the organ responsible for cleaning up your bloodstream and detoxifying your body. A good multivitamin, along with a few other key supplements, will give your liver additional support. That way, your busy liver can spend less time struggling to process toxins and more time metabolizing fat instead!

The best supplements for liver support contain artichoke extract, broccoli concentrate, curcumin, methionine, methylfolate, silymarin, taurine, alpha lipoic acid, n-acetylosteine, and B12. You can find them at your local health foods stores typically, but ensure that you discuss any new supplement regimen with your physician and your pharmacist first.

MAGNESIUM Recommended Daily Dose: 120–320 mg of magnesium glycinate. (I may use higher levels for specific medical conditions or if someone is very deficient.)

Chromium

Chromium is an essential mineral that is important in carbohydrate metabolism, particularly blood sugar control mechanisms and stability. It helps cells become more sensitive to insulin. It may also help lower cholesterol levels.

Wheat is the primary source of chromium for most Americans. But because 40–70 percent of chromium is lost when whole-wheat flour is refined into white flour, deficiencies are not uncommon. In addition, a diet high in refined sugars can cause you to excrete more chromium through your urine.

CROMIUM Recommended Daily Dose: 100–400 mcg

Folic Acid (Folate)

Folate, or folic acid, helps increase your energy levels, as well as helps with the metabolism of your cells. The most well-known form of folate is folic acid, which was added to our food supply when researchers discovered that neural tube birth defects were drastically reduced once pregnant women received added folic acid through supplements and through fortifying the food supply with folic acid.

Some studies have shown that folate supplementation is associated with a lowered cancer risk—but others show that taking more than 800 mcg of folic acid daily is linked to an *increased* risk of certain cancers, like colon cancer. Although the cancer link is still uncertain, it is known that up to 60 percent of Americans have genetic variations that prevent folic acid from being metabolized into its active form, called methylfolate. Perhaps the incomplete metabolism of synthetic folic acid is what causes potentially adverse effects.

FOLIC ACID (FOLATE) Recommended Daily Dose: 400–800 mcg sourced from methylfolate (5-methyltetra-hydrofolate)

Methylfolate is the best folate for weight loss. It is easy to metabolize, and because it is water-soluble, it is unlikely to cause any toxicity.

Alpha Lipoic Acid

ALPHA LIPOIC ACID
Recommended Daily Dose:
100–300 mg (higher if you
are diabetic; discuss with your
physician)

All of your cells have a boundary membrane to keep what's inside the cell separate from what's outside it. Alpha lipoic acid helps maintain the proper shape and function of this membrane, and this in turn helps your cells use the glucose they need more efficiently—important to control the **MD Factor**.

Alpha lipoic acid is also extremely helpful for repairing damaged and aged cell membranes, promoting healthy vascular and blood vessel function, and protecting nerve cells from damage.

It's best to take alpha lipoic acid as a vegetarian capsule, without any added fillers or binders.

Cinnamon

CINNAMON Recommended
Daily Dose: teaspoon, in food
or as 100 mg capsule

Several studies have shown that adding as little as ½ teaspoon of cinnamon to your diet daily can improve the **MD Factor**. In addition to improving your body's blood sugar response, cinnamon can also lower your triglycerides, blood pressure, and LDL cholesterol.

EGCG

The word "antioxidant" is used a lot in healthcare and skin care, but many people don't know what it actually is. An antioxidant is a scavenger of damaging free radicals. A free radical is a molecule with an imbalance of electrons. Free radicals can wreak havoc on your cell membranes, causing the damaged cells to age prematurely, and on your DNA, possibly leading to cancer.

Epigallocatechin gallate (EGCG) is a powerhouse antioxidant. Not only does it stop free radicals from forming, but it helps protect your DNA. Powerful enough to reduce inflammation in the walls of blood vessels by preventing the buildup of plaque, EGCG also blocks blood vessel cells from dividing into tumor cells.

One of the best sources of EGCG is green tea. Green tea is a superfood that's particularly loaded with catechins, plant metabolites with antioxidant capabilities—and EGCG is what you could call a supercatechin!

The antioxidant activity of green tea is twenty-five to one hundred times more potent than vitamin C and vitamin E.

EGCG Recommended Daily Dose: At least 10–50 mg of mixed catechins, normally found in 2 cups of green tea. Supercharge it with lemon or other citrus juice, as the acid helps the catechins survive your digestive tract much more successfully. If you don't like the taste of green tea, take a supplement containing green tea extracted from the leaf. Make sure to get no less than 100 mg, which provides approximately 23 mg of EGCG.

- A cup of green tea provides around 10–40 mg of polyphenols (plant antioxidants) and has antioxidant activity greater than a serving of broccoli, spinach, carrots, or strawberries.

- The EGCG in green tea improves your cardiovascular health by lowering LDL or "bad" cholesterol and can begin to lower your blood pressure after only three weeks of use.

- It can break down fat tissue and promote weight loss by helping to control and regulate insulin production. This is especially important if you have the **MD Factor**. In one study, those taking green tea supplements saw their waistlines and their fasting blood sugar levels decrease, and they lost an average of thirty pounds, while those taking a placebo only lost an average of eleven. That's a big difference.

N-Acetylcysteine

N-acetylcysteine (NAC) is a potent amino acid that functions as an antioxidant and free radical scavenger. This is extremely important, because fat tissue sends out inflammatory chemicals. This inflammation causes all kinds of problems, and the one most people tend to notice is belly bloat.

NAC has many other health benefits. It can improve symptoms of polycystic ovarian syndrome; helps remove toxic heavy metals such as mercury and lead from your body; enhances nail growth and makes nails less brittle; keeps the membranes of the respiratory system moist, which lessens irritation from dry air, dust, and pollutants; and helps your immune system to do its job properly in your respiratory tract. In addition, your body uses NAC to create glutathione, your body's most prevalent and important molecule for detoxification. Glutathione forms a complex with substances such as pesticides and pollutants to stabilize them and remove them from your body.

Omega-3s

There are several omega-3 fatty acids. One is ALA, or alpha linolenic acid, and it's a component of plant foods such as walnuts and chia seeds. Since our body cannot produce omega-3 fatty acids, we have to consume them. Another important omega-3 fatty acid is gamma linolenic acid, or GLA, which is found in foods such as avocados, evening primrose oil, and sunflower seeds. Both ALA and GLA have powerful anti-inflammatory properties and can be helpful for repairing the cellular damage that occurs with the **MD Factor**.

Fish consume these same types of omega-3s and convert them a step further into more bioavailable forms called EPA and DHA. Consuming these healthful fats on a regular basis can reduce inflammation and blood clots and lower your triglyceride levels. They also help regulate vasodilation as well as vasoconstriction (the expansion and contraction of your blood vessels). All of these things together reduce your risk of developing heart disease. Taking an omega-3 supplement of EPA and DHA can also lower blood pressure, lower triglyceride levels, and decrease the risk of sudden death from arrhythmia (irregular heart beat) in people with heart disease, which is why the American Heart Association recommends that adults with those conditions take omega-3 supplements daily.

Eating fish is a good way to get omega-3s, but farm-raised fish such as salmon have lower levels than wild-caught fish. And many people don't like fish or avoid it due to concerns about mercury or ocean pollutants such as PCBs.

It's important to choose a top-quality fish oil. Make sure the label states clearly that the oil has been tested for purity, guaranteeing that it's free of PCBs, dioxins, and mercury. A good test for fish oil quality is to break the capsule open. If it smells fishy, it is probably rancid, so you should replace it. It's best to store fish oil in the refrigerator and only buy a one-to-two-month supply at a time. Check the expiration dates as well.

Berberine as a Boost

BERBERINE: Recommended Daily Dose 350–500 mg per capsule and slowly increase up to three times a day

Sometimes my patients follow the **MD Factor** Action Plan, take their supplements, and exercise regularly, but their **MD Factor** is stubborn and just doesn't want to let go. When that happens, I often recommend berberine, an herbal insulin sensitizer that is widely used in China in the treatment of type 2 diabetes.

What Kind of Vitamin or Mineral Capsule Is Best?

I prefer vitamins and minerals in vegetarian capsules. This dissolves quickly and readily, allowing the supplements to be more readily absorbed by your body. Tablets normally have a coating that makes it a little harder for your body to digest, and many of them contain fillers and binders, which are needed to hold the tablet together or to stabilize the ingredients. These fillers and binders provide no health benefits, and some people have sensitivities to them.

A Note of Caution

The recommendations in this chapter are prescribed to my patients while under my care. Always consult your physician before beginning any type of vitamin or supplement.

CHAPTER 8

The Exercise You Don't Need—Yet

What was that?" I can hear you say. "I don't need to exercise to lose weight?" This may be hard to believe, but if you are currently not exercising regularly, don't start—yet. The reason is simple: research shows that changing your diet is much more important than changing your exercise level when you want to lose weight. Or, to put it in the terms I've been using, changing your diet to have it work with your metabolism is much more important than changing your exercise.

Think about it. You've read in the preceding chapters about how your metabolism falls if you don't eat adequate protein throughout the day, and how if you have the **MD Factor** and eat too many carbohydrates, your body stores as fat all the glucose your body can't use right away. This fat-storing metabolism needs to change—and this is the most important objective.

When you want to lose weight, the typical thinking is that you must eat fewer calories. If you eat enough protein to spare your muscles and eat less calories overall, you will lose fat. As you know already, some of my patients have to eat more protein and sometimes even *more* calories than they have been eating, and only then are they able to lose weight.

But what about exercise? Doesn't exercise burn calories?

Of course it does, and exercise is great for overall health and to strengthen your cardiovascular system and muscles. Many of my patients are highly motivated to lose weight, and they want to start the dietary program and get going in the gym or with a trainer. When I test them and find they do have the **MD Factor**, however, I ask them to hold off on the exercise at first and focus their energy on the meal plan to defeat the **MD Factor**.

Because the **MD Factor** Action Plan requires a change in eating habits and a bit more planning than most people are used to, I want everyone to concentrate on getting their meal plans correct first. Usually after about three weeks on the **MD Factor** Action Plan, everything clicks, and the new way of eating has become a fabulous new habit. Other patients need a slightly longer adjustment time; their lives are complicated and they need a little more time to work out the meal planning, snack planning, and food preparation. And some patients who are very overweight need to lose at least twenty or thirty pounds before they can resolve some of the physical issues that make exercise difficult for them.

I have patients in wheelchairs or with injuries and health conditions that preclude them from exercising, and they *still* are able to lose weight simply by following the **MD Factor** Action Plan and taking the supplements you read about in the previous chapter. In fact, you don't need to start exercising when you start your **MD Factor** Action Plan, and you will still lose weight as the result of your much-improved diet.

So, in contrast to what you've doubtless heard umpteen times—that you should start exercising when you want to lose weight—I want you to wait. Focusing on your diet *first* is more important.

For example, if you described yourself to me as a couch potato, and then you start to walk for half an hour every other day, that will become a pretty big time commitment. You may burn 200–300 calories, but if you aren't yet confident about and accustomed to your new meal planning and snacks, you could return home hungry and tired, and reach for a glass of orange juice and a few crackers. If so, you'll be ingesting more calories (of pure sugar!) than you just burned. That is not the kind of exercise routine that will bring you the results you seek.

If, on the other hand, you exercise regularly already, don't stop! You've already found a way to incorporate regular exercise into your daily life, so the only added adjustment for you is the meal plan. You'll soon find that your new way of eating will give you more energy so you can exercise stronger and harder. If so, you can push yourself a little further, but don't make any big changes to your exercise plan yet. Adjust gradually to avoid injury and overdoing it.

Does That Mean You Never Need to Exercise?

Sorry! You *will* lose weight faster when you add exercise to your total **MD Factor** Action Plan. Just make sure you have the meal plan down *first*.

There's a stronger correlation between additional weight loss and regular exercise in men, more so than for women. Many of my male patients have told me that their weight management strategy has always been to go back to the gym when their belts started getting a little tight.

While exercise might not be necessary for initially losing weight, it is mandatory for keeping the weight off once you've lost it.

But even they found that once they develop the **MD Factor,** extra time in the gym isn't enough to shift the weight as easily as before.

Women do lose weight from increasing their exercise, though it may not be as significant as what men experience. But it's still worth doing, because while exercise might not be necessary for initially losing weight, it is mandatory for keeping the weight off once you've lost it.

We All Need to Move More

The technological marvels of modern society have made our lives so much easier in so many ways. You don't have to get up to change the channel on the TV set—just hit a button on the remote. No more walking into the bank or the fast-food restaurant or the gas station—just order from the drive-up window or pay at the pump. No more push lawnmowers or vacuum cleaners—just plug it in and watch the mower self-propel or have a robotic device suck up the dust. No more washing the dishes by hand—load the dishwasher. Why, we don't even have to wait a few more seconds to dial a telephone (remember *that*?).

For example, I drive my kids to school, as do most parents in my Florida community. Back when I was younger, my parents wouldn't have dreamed of giving me a ride to school. I walked to all my schools, and in high school it was over a mile just to get to my bus stop. There was no choice given—I had to do it. My friends and classmates all had to do it. As a result, we burned calories and stayed strong without even thinking about it.

Fast-forward a generation. We now need to think about how to go out of our way to incorporate regular exercise into our lives. It's especially important to incorporate regular exercise into your new **MD Factor** Action Plan lifestyle, because exercise is a very powerful tool for correcting the **MD Factor** and losing weight, and to keep it from coming back.

The Best Exercise for You

Once you get going, you will be amazed at how much better you feel, how much energy you have, and how drastically your appetite can decline with regular exercise. Still, many people understand the benefits of exercise—but the reality of starting is something else entirely.

Here are some tips for beginning your exercise routine:

✔ **Create a music playlist** and make sure your headphones won't fall out of your ears (which can be very frustrating). For some people, this playlist might be soothing, with calming tunes to walk to so you can unwind after a busy day. This is hugely beneficial for stress relief and clearing your system of cortisol, the hormone released by your adrenal glands when you are stressed. For others, more energetic and invigorating music is motivating and empowering. There's nothing like dance music to really get your mood up and help drive you to push yourself just a little bit harder.

✔ **Invite a friend along to go with you.** Workout buddies are terrific, as you keep each other motivated. Be sure, however, to have a backup plan in case your workout buddy has to cancel. A good playlist of music you love can help replace the conversation you were planning to have.

✔ **Ignore everyone else.** If you have a membership at the gym, make sure you really feel comfortable there. Ignore everyone else. The worst thing you can do when in a gym is compare yourself to others, leaving yourself feeling inadequate, uncoordinated, or frustrated.

✔ **Wear a pedometer all day.** Try tracking how many steps you've taken. Write down the results to track your progress. Aim to increase your steps by two hundred each day. Ten thousand steps a

Once you get going, you will be amazed at how much better you feel, how much energy you have, and how drastically your appetite can decline.

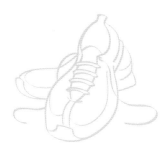

day, which equates to five miles, can provide drastic improvements in your health.

✔ **Morning exercise tends to produce the best results** for fat burn because you have been fasting while sleeping and your body is already breaking down fat to provide glucose to your body. This might help motivate you when the alarm goes off! I have also found that exercising first thing allows you to get it done before all the other many responsibilities and commitments of your day get piled on.

✔ **Prepare the night before.** If your workout time is first thing in the morning, set out your workout clothes and shoes before you go to sleep. As soon as you see them, change right away and get going rather than hitting the snooze button! If your workout time is in the afternoon, change into your workout clothes right after work. You'll be more likely to go if your tennis shoes are already on—and if you don't change, you're more likely to skip the workout. Grab a water bottle and do not make a detour to your home first. Once you arrive there, it's too tempting to find other tasks to do that are seemingly more pressing than exercise.

✔ **Schedule your exercise.** Treat it like a doctor's appointment—in other words, one that you are not going to cancel without serious repercussions!

✔ **Start with a small, doable amount of time.** Even five minutes is much better than zero minutes. Increase your exercise time very slowly, too. For example, if you're watching a one-hour TV show, do some exercising during the commercials. Without even realizing it, you'll have done about twenty minutes' worth of workouts each hour.

✔ **Record each time and for how long you exercise.** Make a graph and post it somewhere visible in the house so you can see how much you are doing and how well you're progressing.

✔ **Hire a pro.** If you can afford it, I recommend hiring a personal trainer for at least a few sessions. Interview potential candidates first to be sure you'll click with their personality and training style. A certified trainer will teach you the right way to exercise, which is especially important for anyone starting a weight training program. (Believe me, most people lifting weights in my local gym are using incorrect form; not only is this ineffective training, but they're putting themselves at risk for injuries). A good trainer will motivate you in the right way and keep you going through the entire length of your session. If finances are an issue, try hiring a trainer for a small group, as you'll still get personalized attention.

✔ **Don't overdo it.** Don't try to run a mile if you haven't run one before, or if it's been years since you did. Your muscles need to get strong first. If you overcommit, chances are high that you will either get hurt, get frustrated, or get angry that you're not progressing the way you think you should. Setting much smaller goals and then achieving them will be much more satisfying and productive.

The Best Forms of Exercise

The best type of exercise is the exercise that gets your heart beating with a smile on your face. In other words, the best type of exercise is the exercise that you really like and that you will keep on doing.

My Own Exercise Routine

Exercise for me is not a chore or something I have to get done. It's my much-needed time for me, and it's important not only for my health but for my family members to see how vital it is for me to do—so they'll be regular exercisers, too.

I've always loved to exercise at the end of the day as a way to de-stress. It helped me get through some rigorous years in medical school where I had to sit in over-air-conditioned classrooms or lecture halls for up to ten hours a day. Getting my body moving helped me clear my head, and it helped me get back to my studies later in the evening.

After I was a practicing physician and my children were born, exercising in the evening became impossible. I wanted to spend time with my little ones, especially as I hadn't seen them all day. And there was dinner to be made, baths to run, and homework to check. If I took the time to exercise in the evening, our entire family routine would come crashing down!

I needed to transition to exercising first thing in the morning. While I don't always love getting up at 5:00 a.m., no one else in my family is up then, and no one else needs me. I can do what I need to do for myself, get my workout done without any interruptions, and start the day invigorated. My routine includes a forty-five-minute spinning class three times a week at the YMCA with great music and an equally great group of supportive people. In addition, I do a forty-five-minute group personal training class that focuses on core strength, balance, and functional training of all the major muscle groups in short one-minute intervals, two to three times a week. This class in particular is marvelously supportive, and the joy I get from being around my fellow exercisers helps when some days we are not fully awake until fifteen minutes into it!

I've found that being consistent with exercise and my own self-care makes me a better mother, wife, doctor, boss, friend, and daughter. Because I have so many responsibilities, I know I can't handle them all effectively and efficiently if I don't make time to take care of myself first.

There are countless ways to get your body moving. Exercise should be *fun*. If you're not having fun, then find a sport or activity that you're going to love. For some people this is solitary running; for others, tennis or basketball or soccer provide not only exercise but also the camaraderie of playing with other teammates. Bike riding, roller skating, walking, jogging, or even throwing a Frisbee can be good ways to get outside and get moving. If you live in a metropolitan area, try taking a spinning class or a beginner yoga or Pilates class. Try martial arts or boxing, as hitting things is a fantastic way to thwack the stress out of your body! Dance classes are extremely effective for strengthening your core muscles and making you feel good about learning a terrific new skill.

Another type of exercise that might be enticing is interval training. This kind of workout puts large demands on your body for short periods of time. Not only isn't there a huge time commitment, but any exercise that requires short bursts of intense energy can help you release natural human growth hormone, which helps build lean muscle tissue and speed up your metabolic rate.

Don't forget to add strength training to your regular cardiovascular exercise routine. It's best to do a workout with weights at least twice a week. And regular weight training adds lean muscle mass, which helps raise your metabolism. This is especially good for women, as it helps keep bones and muscles strong. And because women have smaller amounts of muscle mass to begin with, adding lean muscle definitely helps lessen the **MD Factor**.

So next time you're exhausted, tell yourself that there's no downside to exercise—aside from doing too much too fast, which could lead to getting hurt. Start slow, write it all down, gradually increase your workout time, and challenge yourself. Before you know it, your fatigue will be gone, you'll be amazed at your toned muscles, and you'll be feeling great.

I've found that being consistent with exercise and my own self-care makes me a better mother, wife, doctor, boss, friend, and daughter.

When to Eat When You're Exercising Regularly

Doctors and trainers often disagree about the best time to eat when exercising. Some exercise specialists insist on exercising on an empty stomach in order to take advantage of the fact that your body has been breaking down fat for fuel, and then eating something afterward like a protein shake or a meal. Other research shows that drinking a protein shake before you exercise causes muscle-building amino acids to be delivered straight into your bloodstream, and fewer amino acids are lost in the process of protein turnover.

While differences in the timing of eating and exercise may matter for serious athletes, I find it makes no clinical difference for my patients.

I recommend having a light protein shake before weight training workouts if that is convenient. I don't recommend having a large full meal before a workout, as blood flow that needs to go to your muscles for exercise gets diverted to your stomach when you're digesting a lot of food.

The *composition* of what you eat in the hours before and after exercise is what matters the most. You need to replace the amino acids broken down by exercise by eating enough protein in your meals. When you eat carbohydrates, you want the complex, slowly digested type such as vegetables, fruit, nuts, or small amounts of whole grains—exactly what you'll find on the **MD Factor** Action Plan!

What to Do When You're Just Too Tired to Move

If you are constantly tired—and *way* too tired to exercise—guess what? That's the best time to exercise! A mere ten minutes more of exercise each day can replenish your energy levels and beat the blahs better than a ten-minute sprawl on the sofa, as tempting as that may be.

Exercise gets your blood flowing. Even something as simple as a leisurely stroll can boost your energy levels by about 20 percent. Light workouts fight fatigue even more, while also boosting your mood and improving your stress load and your health. Since exercise releases endorphins, the feel-good hormones, it makes you feel good, and it can improve your memory, sex drive, and, best of all, help you reverse the **MD Factor**.

CHAPTER 9

The Alcohol You Need to Watch

Drinking alcohol is part of our culture. Good or bad—and there are both pluses and minuses to drinking—alcohol consumption and the marketing of alcohol as a seductive, pleasurable pastime are not going anywhere. Just look to the failure of Prohibition at the beginning of the twentieth century for an example!

If you do drink, however, it's very important to understand what alcohol does to your body, so you can make an informed decision about how much will give you potential health benefits and how too much can make you seriously ill and wreak havoc on your **MD Factor**. It's very easy to get confused, what with all the seemingly contradictory reports that come out about drinking. Is moderate drinking good for you? What's moderate? What is too much? Does it increase your risk of cancer or help prevent the disease? Likewise with heart disease. And what about the studies that have shown that men and women who drink moderately often weigh less than those who don't drink at all?

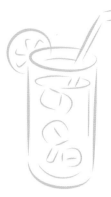

Drinking wine in moderation, particularly red wine, has been shown to decrease your risk of heart attacks. It can also lower your blood sugar. Having a drink can also be a pleasurable way to de-stress and unwind, or to savor a relaxing meal with friends.

What Is Moderate Alcohol Consumption?

It's very important to understand what moderate consumption really means, as it is a much lower level than many people assume.

For men, a maximum of ten glasses of wine (or the equivalent) per week is considered a moderate alcohol intake. Men who have three drinks each day, seven days a week, are doubling the recommended amount.

For women, five glasses of wine (or the equivalent) per week is considered a moderate alcohol intake. Women's livers are much smaller than men's, which makes it harder to detoxify higher alcohol levels. This is why women can get intoxicated more quickly if they have the same amount of alcohol as men.

A standard drink is defined as:

✔ **12 ounces** of beer
✔ **5 ounces** of wine
✔ **1.5 ounces** of spirits (vodka, whiskey, etc.)

I'm sure you've already realized from looking at this list that many drinks you're served in a social setting or at home contain much more than one serving. You can unwittingly be drinking more servings than you intended in one glass of wine, if the glass is large.

Some of my female patients are absolutely shocked when I discuss this with them. They're smart and savvy and are often brilliant at deciphering food labels and understanding fat and calorie content so they can buy the best food for their families. They're pros at counting calories for food. When it comes to alcoholic beverages, however, they often falter, because they just don't know how to count those types of calories.

For example, if a woman has two glasses of wine every night, she's drinking an average of fourteen drinks per week. That is almost three times the recommended moderate consumption level of five drinks. And those calories quickly add up.

The Alcohol Calorie Count

Alcohol is not a nutrient. It's a toxin. Whenever you drink alcohol, it first goes to your liver to be detoxified and is then processed as sugar. This is why drinking alcohol can make it so hard for you to lose weight.

Each gram of alcohol contains seven calories (remember, each gram of fat contains nine calories).* Patients of mine who would never dream of eating cheesecake are shocked when I tell them that drinking two glasses of wine is the equivalent of eating a small piece of that dessert! Your body doesn't care if the calories are liquid or solid—they're still calories.

In other words, each serving of alcohol contains approximately the same calories as 10 grams of fat. That translates to about 100 calories for each serving. Add in the sugar from the grapes in wine, the mixers in your margarita, or the additives in beer, and if you have a large drink—or more than one—these calories very quickly add up.

Part of the problem is that, in general, your stomach registers calories from food much more quickly than it registers calories from liquids. It's easy to drink a lot of lemonade or soda or wine and not feel full at all, even if you've just put 800 calories into your body. When you do the math, those liquid calories really do count.

Alcoholic Beverage	Calories
4 oz. martini	275
12 oz. daiquiri	675
12 oz. margarita	750
5 oz. red wine	125
5 oz. white wine	120
10 oz. Long Island ice tea	580
12 oz. piña colada	655
12 oz. regular beer	145
12 oz. light beer	110
1½ oz. vodka with cranberry juice	150

*A standard drink contains 14 grams of alcohol.

Why Drinking Alcohol Makes It So Hard to Lose Weight

Having a few drinks isn't just about ingesting additional calories you underestimated. Alcohol has many effects on your body:

Toxicity

As I mentioned previously, your body treats alcohol more like a toxin than like a nourishing food. This explains why patients of mine who were eating only about 1,000 calories each day—including alcohol—still couldn't lose weight. As you know, your liver is the organ responsible for ridding your body of toxins. It also needs to be able to detoxify and breakdown fat tissue. Whenever you drink, your liver makes the breakdown of the alcohol a priority. As long as your liver is busy detoxifying alcohol, it can't focus on metabolizing fat tissue as efficiently.

MD Factor trigger

Many of my patients have told me that having a drink or two helps them fall asleep easily, but then they often wake up after only a few hours and can't fall back asleep. They're exhausted and out of sorts the next day. This happens because alcohol lowers blood sugar levels. When you have the **MD Factor**, you see big surges in insulin after you eat or drink, but then when your cells finally do get the sugar they need, your blood sugar levels drop into relative hypoglycemia. Your body perceives this as so stressful and potentially life-threatening that it wakes you up. Even if you do fall back asleep, you'll probably wake up again an hour or two later as this cycle repeats itself.

Lowered inhibitions

One of the reasons it's enjoyable to drink is that it's relaxing and often lowers inhibitions. This is fine if you need to unwind, but not so fine when you are in a restaurant, where after the first drink that bread basket suddenly looks amazingly tempting—and after the second or third, dessert doesn't sound so bad. Don't forget the coffee with cream and sugar. Skip the wine or cocktails and it's easier to skip all of those dinnertime extras.

Hormonal effects

I often joke with my perimenopausal or menopausal patients that the easiest way to trigger a hot flash is to have a drink and then eat some simple carbohydrates, like a bowl of pasta, white rice, or a baked potato. Declining hormonal levels already make blood sugar regulation more difficult, and having a drink or two can become the tipping point for hot flashes.

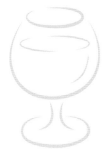

Water retention and dehydration

Alcohol causes water retention, leaving you bloated and puffy and feeling uncomfortable. In what might seem like a contradiction, alcohol can dehydrate you at the same time.

Serious medical issues

Excessive, chronic alcohol consumption can lead to heart disease, strokes, cancer (particularly breast, liver, pancreas, esophagus, and throat), cirrhosis of the liver, and dementia. Alcohol addiction can kill you.

Bottom line

You don't need to stop drinking if you enjoy it—and if you can control the amount of alcohol you consume rather than it controlling you. When you're trying to lose weight, it's a good idea to limit your servings to one to two drinks per week for women and two to four drinks per week for men. You can use measuring cups when you're at home, and that will give you a good idea of the right amount to drink in social settings.

CHAPTER 10

The Artificial Sugars You Need to Watch

We've all heard the advice: to lose weight, choose diet soda, pick low-calorie foods, and go for low-carb drinks. Food marketers have responded to public demand and now cram artificial sweeteners in countless products, seemingly every bar, shake, cereal, or beverage on grocery shelves. It's simple: artificial sweeteners reduce calories while maintaining a sweet taste, right? With our nation's epidemic of obesity, how could that be so bad?

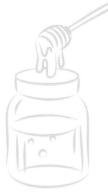

To Be—or Not to Be—Artificially Sweet

Artificial sweeteners aren't necessarily bad, although there have been contradictory studies about whether they can cause cancer or other problems in research studies using animals. The more immediate problem is that there's no good answer about how artificial sweeteners affect your metabolism.

For example, an analysis of health data from a large number of nurses followed for twenty-five years showed no weight gain for those who drank beverages with artificial sweeteners. Other small, short-term trials show that drinking diet sodas instead of sugar-sweetened beverages reduces weight gain or increases weight loss in controlled settings. Another study showed that normal-weight children who consumed artificially sweetened beverages had decreased weight gain compared to children who drank sugar-sweetened beverages.

On the other hand, there have also been studies that show that people who use artificial sweeteners are more likely to be overweight and have many of the diseases caused by the **MD Factor**, like diabetes and heart disease. It was unclear from the studies if the artificial sweeteners caused the weight gain, or if people who are overweight to begin with use more products with artificial sweeteners than people without a weight problem.

However, recent studies from the Washington School of Medicine have shown that artificial sweeteners can have a powerful effect on insulin levels and, unfortunately, on blood glucose levels as well. One study looked at seventeen very overweight people (100 pounds or more overweight) who didn't consume any artificial sweeteners and were free from diabetes. Volunteers were given one of two things prior to a glucose challenge test: either a glass of water or a drink made with the artificial sweetener sucralose (Splenda). The researchers wanted to discover if drinking sucralose before a glucose challenge test would affect insulin or blood sugar levels. Each volunteer was tested twice, first just by drinking just water, and then a week later with just a sucralose beverage.

The results were very surprising. Compared to water only, the sucralose drink caused approximately a 20 percent increase in peak insulin levels, creating a higher peak plasma glucose concentration. As you know, higher insulin and glucose levels both stimulate and aggravate the **MD Factor**.

Researchers suspected that our taste buds might be responsible. Artificial sweeteners such as sucralose interact with receptors on your tongue, which in turn give your brain a signal that you're consuming something sweet. But your body doesn't necessarily know if what you've just consumed is calorie-free or not, so it prepares for the oncoming arrival of sugar. When this happens, your body never really gets the sugar it thinks is coming. You can see how this may affect your appetite—it leaves you wanting more.

Scientists already know that digestive hormones can be released just by seeing food; a commercial for a juicy steak or doughnut can cause even the most self-controlled of us to salivate a little. The same thing can happen with tasting something sweet. Signals from our tongue get sent to our digestive organs, and these organs react, of course—particularly your pancreas, where insulin is produced and released. In other words, digestive hormones are triggered even when you consume a very low dose of artificial sweeteners. With regard to sucralose, this happens at a dose as low as 48 mg, which is about what you would find in a single 1-gram packet of Splenda. The bottom line is that even small amounts of artificial sweeteners can play tricks on your body, causing it to overrespond to signals from your taste buds. And there may be some evidence that this effect can actually cause weight gain—some studies that

There's no good answer about how artificial sweeteners affect your metabolism.

Skip the diet sodas, which have no nutritional benefit at all, and eat real food.

have looked into artificial sweeteners' ability to help consumers limit their calories each day found that these artificial sweeteners made people gain weight in some settings.

Bear in mind that the most significant source of artificial sweeteners in the American diet comes from diet beverages, which are often consumed in place of food. For example, many of my patients have told me that they drink four or five Diet Cokes a day instead of eating breakfast and lunch, and only eat dinner. They're trying to restrict their calories, and they have diet sodas to try to curb their hunger. Often the one meal they do eat at dinnertime is not overloaded with calories, containing on average maybe 500–800 calories. But even though their daily caloric intake is very low, they are still overweight. Worse, they often find themselves *gaining* weight.

I grew up in a family with weight problems and have a sweet tooth of my own, so I had used artificial sweeteners for years. I often drank diet sodas to get a sweet taste without adding extra calories, as many women do. As I became more educated about sugar metabolism over the years, I've stopped using artificial sweeteners personally and have been able to maintain my weight without difficulty. I have, it must be said, also gotten into the habit of eating consistent and regular meals, all containing adequate protein and the right mix of healthful carbohydrates and fats that work with my metabolism.

Over the years, my dietitians and I have taught our patients to eat more lean protein, fewer simple carbohydrates, and, of course, fewer simple sugars. But we were not sticklers about avoiding artificial sweeteners, because some patients just needed something sweet and we knew that protein products such as shakes or puddings—even those sweetened with an artificial sweetener—were a better choice than large quantities of simple sugars or no protein at all. Many of my patients have found that protein shakes and puddings are a useful tool for them as they correct their **MD Factor**, as they're some of the lowest-calorie ways to take in lean protein. They're also quick and convenient when you're working or traveling and the ability to prepare or order a meal with adequate lean protein is challenging. (It's much harder to carry a few slices of turkey breast in your purse than a protein bar!) I knew it was often much more important that these patients lose their extra pounds at first than to watch the amount of artificial sweetener they were ingesting. But because I do worry about the effect of artificial sweeteners on the **MD Factor**, my team and I are always looking for new protein products without artificial sweeteners to add to our recommended foods and products. (You can see an updated list at **www.MDFactorBook.com**.)

My advice is to skip the diet sodas, which have no nutritional benefit at all, and eat real food. If it is very hard to lose weight, though, protein products with artificial sweeteners could be a useful tool to get the protein you need without too many calories.

Grilled chicken with red pepper sauce and cauliflower mash

THE MD FACTOR ACTION PLAN

CHAPTER 11

The MD Factor Daily Action Plan

The best way to reverse the **MD Factor** is to change the way you feed your cells. They need lots of energy-rich protein and far fewer carbohydrates, especially grains, starches, and sugars.

Symptoms of the **MD Factor** can resolve very quickly once you start eating on a meal plan designed to improve it—usually after only a few days to a few weeks. Most people find that their cravings go away after the first few days, and they are no longer hungry. Obviously, it's much easier to lose weight when you're no longer craving sugar and carbohydrates.

What to Expect When You Start the **MD Factor** Action Plan

MD Factor Action Plan Goals

✔ Increase lean protein intake so that your body gets what it needs and can enter a fat-burning mode.

✔ Reduce your carbohydrate intake so that your body taps into its supply of stored fat.

✔ Accomplish rapid weight loss at the start, so that you have the incentive to keep going.

✔ Lose your cravings for sugar, sweets, refined carbohydrates, and other foods that trigger the **MD Factor**. Once you've broken the cycle, your body will simply not crave them anymore.

On the detailed meal plans you'll find in this chapter, you'll see that you start your Action Plan with three Reclaim days before moving on to the Transformation, or weight loss, days. You need to follow the plan exactly for maximum results. The Reclaim days are the only part of the meal plan that are really restrictive, and these are undertaken for a reason: to clear your bloodstream of insulin and jump-start your metabolism. My patients have no problem doing this, as nearly all of them find their cravings are so much better after a few days and they know that in three days they will have both more food and a greater variety of food.

As you undoubtedly know, the trouble with most diets is that it's very hard to find one that helps you shed pounds quickly without compromising the nutritional quality of your meals—and ultimately your health and vitality. Literally thousands of people who had the **MD Factor** have been treated at my medical center, and they've gotten results. They lost weight, reversed their **MD Factor**, and feel great.

Eat More to Lose Weight

My dietitians and I are often told that the **MD Factor** Action Plan, with the exception of the Reclaim days, contains too much food. It's usually women who tell us this. We know that many of these women are so used to starving themselves that they think the only way to lose weight is by eating next to nothing. They keep detailed dietary logs meticulously listing their drastically low caloric intakes from their carefully weighed and measured portions. They're distraught because they continue to gain weight, even though the numbers show they should be losing weight. What I explain to them is that the **MD Factor** has altered their metabolism to predominantly store fat. Eating the right balance and volume of nutritious food on the **MD Factor** Action Plan will correct your metabolism, stop you from feeling you need to starve, and allow you to finally start losing weight.

An Overview of the Structure of the Plan

There are three different types of days for you to follow to correct the **MD Factor**.

As I've noted, you start with three Reclaim days. These will clear your bloodstream of insulin and jump-start your metabolism.

Reclaim days are followed by Transformation days, which you will remain on for three and a half weeks. Transformation days are designed to keep your energy level high, your appetite satisfied, and your body locked into a fat-burning mode.

The only difference between the Reclaim days and Transformation days is the amount of carbohydrates you can eat. The protein and fat requirements remain the same.

The Transformation days are followed by the Stabilization days, where you'll be eating more carbs for six days. These six Stabilization days are then followed by one Reclaim day. This stabilization cycle is repeated twice, over a two-week time frame.

You may have reached your goal weight at the end of this six-week cycle, depending on how strong your **MD Factor** is and how much weight you needed to lose. If you have made great progress and want to lose more body fat, this cycle can be repeated with up to four weeks of Transformation days followed by the Stabilization phase again. This can be repeated as many times as is necessary to arrive at your goal weight.

3
RECLAIM DAYS

25
TRANSFORMATION DAYS

6
STABILIZATION DAYS

Your Weight Loss Calendar

The easiest way to keep track of your **MD Factor** Action Plan schedule is with a calendar. Use this template to help you with your schedule.

Reclaim Day	Reclaim days, for insulin sensitizing: less than 60 grams of carbs
Transformation Day	Transformation days, for weight loss: between 60 and 100 grams of carbs
Stabilization Day	Stabilization days, for weight maintenance: between 100 and 150 grams of carbs

Monday	Tuesday	Wednesday	Thursday	Friday	Saturday	Sunday
Day 1 R	Day 2 R	Day 3 R	Day 4 T	Day 5 T	Day 6 T	Day 7 T
Day 8 T	Day 9 T	Day 10 T	Day 11 T	Day 12 T	Day 13 T	Day 14 T
Day 15 T	Day 16 T	Day 17 T	Day 18 T	Day 19* T	Day 20 T	Day 21 T
Day 22 T	Day 23 T	Day 24 T	Day 25 T	Day 26* T	Day 27 T	Day 28 T
Day 29 S	Day 30 S	Day 31 S	Day 32 S	Day 33* S	Day 34 S	Day 35 R
Day 36 S	Day 37 S	Day 38 S	Day 39 S	Day 40* S	Day 41 S	Day 42 R
Day 43 T	Day 44 T	Day 45 T	Day 46 T	Day 47* T	Day 48 T	Day 49 T
Day 50 T	Day 51 T	Day 52 T	Day 53 T	Day 54* T	Day 55 T	Day 56 T
Day 57 T	Day 58 T	Day 59 T	Day 60 T	Day 61* T	Day 62 T	Day 63 T
Day 64 T	Day 65 T	Day 66 T	Day 67 T	Day 68* T	Day 69 T	Day 70 T

*Represents a structured break from the program, called "My Night." Our research shows that this enables you to make healthy choices on your own.

*The **MD Factor** Diet*

The **MD Factor** Plan Cheat Sheet

3 RECLAIM DAYS
Women: 120 grams of protein, less than 60 grams of net carbs, 30 grams of fat
Men: 140 grams of protein, less than 60 grams of net carbs, 40 grams of fat

25 TRANSFORMATION DAYS
Women: 120 grams of protein, between 60–100 grams of net carbs, 30 grams of fat
Men: 140 grams of protein, between 60–100 grams of net carbs, 40 grams of fat

6 STABILIZATION DAYS
Women: 120 grams of protein, 100–150 grams of net carbs, 30–40 grams of fat
Men: 140 grams of protein, 100–150 grams of net carbs, 40–60 grams of fat

1 RECLAIM DAY
Women: 120 grams of protein, less than 60 grams of net carbs, 30 grams of fat
Men: 140 grams of protein, less than 60 grams of net carbs, 40 grams of fat

6 STABILIZATION DAYS
Women: 120 grams of protein, 100–150 grams of net carbs, 30–40 grams of fat
Men: 140 grams of protein, 100–150 grams of net carbs, 40–60 grams of fat

1 RECLAIM DAY
Women: 120 grams of protien, less than 60 grams of net carbs, 30 grams of fat
Men: 140 grams of protein, less than 60 grams of net carbs, 40 grams of fat

RESUME TRANSFORMATION DAYS FOR 28 DAYS
Women: 120 grams of protein, 60–100 grams of net carbs, 30 grams of fat
Men: 140 grams of protein, 60–100 grams of net carbs, 40 grams of fat

Continue this cycle until you reach your goal weight. At this point, you will add in more healthy fats and more healthy carbohydrates as you successfully create the new you.

The Prep: Before You Begin

Clean Out the Refrigerator

Look in your refrigerator. Get rid of any old or expired foods. We all have these.

Section off a part of the refrigerator that will be designated for your foods. Other members of the family *must* ask if you want to share any of your designated food, before they eat it!

If there are foods in the fridge that typically tempt you, put them in the back or on the bottom shelves, where they are less visible or accessible. For example, put sugar-sweetened jams, jellies, ketchup, rich dressings, butter, and sweets on a separate shelf for others to use.

Discard or finish off open bottles of wine. Remove the unopened ones and put them away in a cupboard or bar. Avoid drinking any alcohol until you have mastered the Action Plan and have learned how to integrate these items into your diet.

Clean Out the Freezer

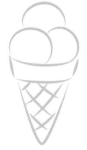

Give away or discard temptations such as ice cream, waffles, candy, ice pops, frozen potatoes, or frozen bread items. If other members of your household eat these foods, designate a freezer space just for you.

Put Aunt Jane's homemade cookies in a freezer bag at the bottom of the freezer. Do this with any special dessert item that you love and that you will be able to eat once you have lost weight, but don't go out and buy those desserts now for later.

Fill your section of the freezer with frozen veggies, chicken breasts, and fish.

Clean Out the Pantry and Cupboards

Partition your pantry and cupboards into spaces for "usable" and "unusable" foods. Try to find a space that is hard to reach for the unusable items.

In the usable section, stock canned tuna, salmon, sardines, and chicken, along with canned veggies such as beets, artichoke hearts, green beans, tomatoes, and your other favorites. In the unusable section, place your baking supplies, such as flour, sugar, and oils.

Give away or discard sugared Jell-O; cake, brownie, cornbread, pancake, or cookie mixes; crackers and cookies; potato chips, cheese curls, and corn chips; boxed macaroni and cheese; packaged rice or side dishes; and fruit chews, candy, and chocolate. These might be tasty, but they are nothing more than highly processed and empty carbohydrates and sugars.

In the unusable section, also put fruit juice and drink mixes. Avoid them until you have mastered the Action Plan and have learned how to integrate these items into your diet.

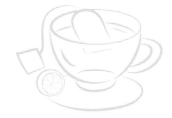

The Day Before You Start:
Getting Ready for Your Action Plan

✔ Drink plenty of water today. Try to drink eight glasses, or four 16-ounce bottles. (Coffee and diet soda don't count, as these are diuretics and deplete your body of water.)

✔ Brew some green tea and try a cup hot and a cup iced, to see what you prefer. I personally like organic jasmine green tea.

✔ If you are already exercising, keep it up! If you are not currently exercising, we will not add anything just yet, as described in Chapter 8.

✔ Take your daily multivitamin (see Chapter 7).

✔ Try to limit yourself to no more than two cups of coffee per day. If you are drinking lots more than this, gradually decrease it and replace it with refreshing water.

✔ Stock up on items you can eat.

✔ Check your calendar for upcoming special events such as birthdays, anniversaries, graduations, and important business meetings or dinners. Prepare for these by mentally agreeing to stick with your program as best you can. The **MD Factor** Action Plan allows you to eat free meals at times that we call "My Nights", so you might want to save those for your important events.

✔ Read through the meal plans later in this chapter. It will be a lot easier to follow the **MD Factor** Daily Action Plan closely at first, so you can get used to it without having to spend any extra time planning what to eat.

MD Factor Stimulant Foods That Increase Your MD Factor and Make Your Metabolism Store Fat

These foods should be eliminated, even if they are whole-grain. Their carbohydrate counts are all too high for your metabolism right now.

Starches

- Bagels
- Bread or rolls
- Cereals
- Corn
- Cornbread
- Cornstarch
- Crackers
- Croissants
- Flour
- Granola
- Muffins
- Noodles
- Pancakes
- Pita bread
- Potatoes
- Rice
- Taco shells
- Tortillas
- Hamburger or hot dog buns

Sweets

- Candy
- Doughnuts
- Corn syrup
- Dried fruits
- Ice cream
- Fruit juice
- Italian ice, sherbet
- Jam or jelly
- Honey
- Molasses
- Pastries
- Pie
- Cookies
- Pudding
- Sweetened Sodas
- Sugar (white, brown)
- Frozen Yogurt
- High-fructose corn syrup

Others

- Corn chips
- Egg rolls
- Sausage
- Hot dogs
- Pizza
- Potato chips
- Popcorn
- Pretzels
- Waffles
- Margarine
- Fried food
- Rice cakes
- French fries
- Fruit juice
- Lemonade

Ready to Start

IMPORTANT NOTE:
If you have diabetes, severe migraine headaches, or heart disease, or if you are over sixty-five years old, I recommend you skip the Reclaim days entirely and begin your meal plan with Transformation Days. If you have another serious medical condition, please get your physician's approval before starting the **MD Factor** Meal Plan.

Reclaim Days

The Reclaim days are designed to jump-start your metabolism. The carbohydrate level on these days is very low. In our office we instruct our patients to keep their carbohydrate intake to below 50–60 grams per day. I will not ask you to keep track of your grams of carbohydrates, because if you follow the template for these three days, you will not exceed this carbohydrate level.

It is very important to be aware that this is three days of a restrictive diet. It is not meant to be followed for any longer than this. It is designed to clear your bloodstream of high insulin levels, which is very effective for reducing cravings. After you complete these three days, you never need to do three days again except for special circumstances (see the sidebar "What Should I Do If I Get Off Track?" on page 168). In the stabilization phase you will do one Reclaim day each week for two weeks.

After the first three Reclaim days, you can expect to feel lighter. Most people notice their cravings for carbs and junk food have decreased. Normally, any water weight will drop off during this time as well, as your system clears itself of the high insulin levels that had been circulating in your bloodstream.

As you already learned in Chapter 4, the most important piece of the weight loss puzzle is protein. Without the basis of lean protein to make up the majority of your meals, your metabolism will not begin to regroup and retrain your system to burn fat. This doesn't necessarily mean you must eat more meat. On the contrary—some of my patients are vegetarians, and they do well with the recommended food choices.

To prepare your food, you can broil, bake, boil, barbecue, microwave, roast, or "fry" using a quick spritz of cooking spray. Limit red meat to twice per week.

The ideal serving of protein is 25–35 grams at every meal. This meets the protein threshold you need so that your body can begin absorbing all the amino acids it needs, which helps regulate insulin. It is crucial to hit that 25–35 gram mark at every meal. If you fall short, you may be a lot hungrier, and your body will resist weight loss.

I have listed protein foods into portion sizes that provide 25–35 grams of protein. Some protein foods you can eat alone, such as chicken breast or lean beef. But other protein foods have too much fat to stand alone as your sole source of protein for a meal. For example, most cheeses are on this list. If you were to get 30 grams of protein from cheese, it

A Word about Math

I don't want to make this meal plan an exercise in complicated math. However, doing some simple math really gives you access to keys for metabolism correction. At my office, patients work one-on-one with the same dietitian for several weeks in a row. In these weekly meetings we can instruct and reinforce any concepts about the meal plan that may have been confusing. As a reader of this book, you don't have a specially trained dietitian sitting next to you, but I know you can do it.

In order to be successful, most women need to get close to 25–30 grams of protein at each of three meals and then get another 20–30 grams during the day in snacks. For most men, the protein goal for meals is 25–35 grams and 40–50 grams during the day in snacks or another mini-meal.

would be accompanied by way too much fat. So I suggest some protein combinations that keep fat at reasonable levels but still provide that critical 25–35 grams of protein.

Here's where the math comes in. You can make your own protein food combinations as long as the amounts add up to 25 to 35 grams of protein. Find your own favorite combos—correcting a metabolism dysfunction and losing weight does not require you to have boring or bland food!

The carbohydrate content of Reclaim days is approximately 50–60 grams per day. If you follow the Reclaim day templates in this book, you will not exceed 60 grams per day. Some of my patients really want to monitor their daily carbohydrate intake as well as their protein intake. Just like with the protein, you can calculate your own carb combos.

On the website, **www.MDFactorBook.com**, I list all the approved proteins, carbohydrates, snacks, and condiments with their grams of protein and carbohydrates for the serving sizes shown. This list is continually being updated with new products.

While spices and most condiments will not add too many carbohydrates, sauces and side dishes made from fruits and grains and other starches will. Remember, the Reclaim period lasts only three days. In Part IV, I have included some of the very flavorful Reclaim day meals created for my program by the chefs of bistroMD. Try these if you have a flair for cooking.

Reclaim Days for Women*

Breakfast:	25–30 g protein, vitamin and mineral supplement, 16 oz. water
Snack:	10–15 g protein, 8 oz. water
Lunch:	25–30 g protein, 1–2 cups cooked or raw vegetables, 2 cups salad with approved dressing, 16 oz. water
Snack:	10–15 g protein, 8 oz. water
Dinner:	25–30 g protein, 1–2 cups cooked or raw vegetables, 2 cups salad with approved dressing, 16 oz. water

Reclaim Days for Men*

Breakfast:	25–35 g protein, vitamin and mineral supplement, 16 oz. water
Snack:	10–20 g protein, 8 oz. water
Lunch:	25–35 g protein, 1–2 cups cooked or raw vegetables (see list), 2 cups salad with approved dressing, 16 oz. water
Snack:	10–20 g protein, 8 oz. water
Dinner:	25–35 g protein, 1–2 cups cooked or raw vegetables, 2 cups salad with approved dressing, 16 oz. water
Snack:	10–20 g protein from the approved list

*See lists later in this chapter for types and serving sizes.

The Best & Leanest Protein Meals

Super-Easy Breakfast

Four options, choose one of the following.

Cottage Cheese Mixer
1 cup of 1% or fat-free
cottage cheese with
1–2 tablespoons
sugar-free jelly or
sugar-free syrup

Egg Whites with Sausage
1 cup liquid egg whites
and 2 vegetarian
sausage patties

Greek Yogurt with Bacon
1 cup plain Greek yogurt with
sugar-free syrup,
with a side of 3 slices
Canadian bacon

Energy Smoothie
1 smoothie (30 g protein; look
for a top-quality whey protein
powder or a complete vegan
protein powder without added
sugar) with 1 serving of fruit
(or try different extracts, like
peppermint or hazelnut),
blended with ice

Easy Breakfast

Three options, choose one of the following.

Egg White Omelet
1 cup liquid egg whites
plus 1 oz. light shredded
Mexican cheese, 1 tablespoon
low-fat sour cream,
and 2 tablespoons salsa

Egg Scramble
1 low-carb tortilla
with egg scramble
(½ cup chopped spinach,
diced tomatoes, ¼ cup
reduced-fat feta cheese,
¾ cup liquid egg whites)

English Muffin with Smoked Salmon
1 toasted light English muffin topped with
a mixture of 3 oz. chopped smoked salmon,
1 slice turkey bacon, 2 tablespoons fat-free cream cheese,
1 tablespoon chopped red onion, and 1 tablespoon chopped
cucumber, finished off with a tomato slice
(make extra smoked salmon mixture so you can
have this again the next day)

Super-Easy Lunch

Four options, choose one of the following:

Tuna Salad

One 6-oz. can chunk light tuna in water, drained, on a bed of lettuce and topped with 2 tablespoons light salad dressing (or lemon juice, salt, and pepper)

Chicken Salad

One 4-oz. pouch or can cooked chicken breast, mixed with 1 tablespoon of reduced-fat mayo, 1 teaspoon of relish, and 1 tablespoon lemon juice, rolled up inside large lettuce leaves

Greek Salad

3-oz. sliced deli turkey or chicken breast topped with 1 tablespoon reduced-fat feta cheese, 2 olives (sliced), and a squeeze of lemon, served on a bed of lettuce

Salmon Salad

One 6-oz. can pink salmon in water, drained, mixed with 1 tablespoon whole grain mustard, 1 teaspoon dill, and a splash of lemon juice served on a bed of lettuce

The MD Factor Diet

Easy Lunch

Four options, choose one of the following:

Mexican Wrap

4 oz. lean ground sirloin cooked
with taco seasonings, topped
with 1 tablespoon
sour cream and
3 tablespoons of salsa,
served on a bed of lettuce or
inside a low-carb wrap

Fish with Steamed Vegetables

5 oz. grouper or salmon
with steamed veggies,
topped with lemon juice

Shrimp Salad

Spinach salad topped
with 4–5 large grilled
shrimp and 2 tablespoons
low-fat salad dressing

Italian Chicken Breast

4–5 oz. baked chicken breast
seasoned with Italian herbs,
topped with 2 oz. of marinara
sauce and a sprinkle of
reduced-fat Parmesan cheese,
served with a salad of fresh
green beans

Dinner

Six options, choose one of the following:

Pork with Sauerkraut

4 oz. pork tenderloin
with 1 cup sauerkraut and
1 cup green beans,
accompanied by a
side salad with
2 tablespoons low-fat
salad dressing

Fish with Spinach Salad

4–5 oz. salmon or other fish,
1 cup of yellow squash
with ½ cup red onion,
fresh spinach salad
on the side

Cheesy Chicken

3–4 oz. chicken breast topped
with ¼ cup tomato sauce and
1 slice reduced-fat
provolone cheese,
with steamed zucchini
and a salad

Light Cheeseburger

4 oz. ground beef mixed with
1 teaspoon Worcestershire
sauce, shaped into a patty and
grilled, topped with 1 slice
of low-fat cheese, mustard,
and tomato, with salad and
fresh carrots

Italian Turkey Breast with Vegetables

4 oz. turkey breast or
tenderloin marinated with
¼ cup Italian dressing,
with ½ cup artichoke hearts,
8 asparagus stalks, and
a small side salad

Asian-Inspired Chicken Breast

4–5 oz. chicken breast, diced,
with 2 teaspoons low-sodium
soy sauce, sauteed with
2 sliced carrots, water
chestnuts, and snow peas

EATS—otherwise known as Essential & Tasty Snacks

In order to keep the **MD Factor** at bay and your blood sugar levels stable, it is absolutely essential that you eat every two to three hours. Snacks containing between 10–15 grams of protein (for women) or 10–20 grams (for men) and that are low in carbohydrates are the best way to combat the **MD Factor**.

If you miss a snack, make sure you eat it later, or else it will be a challenge to meet your daily protein goal.

Real Food Protein Choices

Each of these real food protein choices are 10–15 grams of protein and less than 200 calories.

- ¼ cup nuts
- 2 oz. low-fat cheese
- 2 light string cheese
- 6 oz. light Greek yogurt
- ½ cup low-fat cottage cheese
- 1 tablespoon peanut butter on celery stalks
- ½ cup ricotta cheese
- 2 tablespoons light cream cheese on vegetables
- ¼ cup dry roasted edamame
- 1 tablespoon hummus and 1 oz. lean deli meat

Protein Bars

An extremely easy and convenient protein snack is the protein bar. But not just any protein bar—there are some out there that contain more calories than a candy bar! A good guideline for a protein bar is that it should be less than 180 calories for the whole bar and should contain a minimum of 10 grams of protein and ideally no more than 20 grams of carbohydrates. There are many protein bars on the market and more added each week. Some are better than others.

Please note that some people need to watch their intake of protein bars, as they contain more calories and carbohydrates than other snacks such as a protein drink or lean deli meat. I usually recommend no more than one

Please go to **www.MDFactorBook.com** for updated lists of protein bars available.

protein bar per day while trying to correct the **MD Factor** and lose weight. Some of my patients prefer to split a larger protein bar, such as one that contains 20 grams of protein, in half and have a half twice a day.

Some protein bars contain sugar alcohols, which decrease their net carbohydrate count (see Appendix C) but can cause gas and bloating in some people. Other protein bars have high levels of saturated fat.

Common Protein Portions

This chart gives you visual hints that will help you choose proper portion sizes for your proteins. This makes it easy—no scale is needed; just follow the visual hint.

Protein Source	Serving	Protein (g)	Visual Hint
Chicken breast	4–5 oz. cooked	25–30 g	Size and thickness of your palm
Chicken meatballs	4 medium	25–30 g	Golf ball size
Chicken sausage	2 sausages	25–30 g	Size of a hot dog
Lean beef	3 oz. cooked	25–30 g	Size of a computer mouse
Canadian bacon	5 pieces	25–30 g	Diameter of a hockey puck, but thin
Fish	4–5 oz. cooked	25–30 g	Size and thickness of your palm
Pork tenderloin	4–5 oz. cooked	25–30 g	Size and thickness of your palm
Greek yogurt, plain	1 container	18 g	See approved brands
Cheese, low fat	1 slice	6–7 g	2-by-2-inch coaster
Cheese, low fat	2 cubes	6 g	Game dice
Cheese, string, low fat	2 sticks	12 g	Two thick highlighter markers
Deli meat	3 slices	20 g	Deck of cards
Peanut butter	2 tbsp.	9 g	Ping-pong ball
Beef jerky	2 strips	14 g	12-inch ruler

*The **MD Factor** Diet*

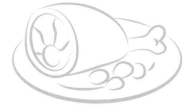

Food Choice	Serving	Protein (g)
Chicken		
Chicken breast, boneless, skinless	4–5 oz.	25–30
Chicken breast, canned	5 oz.	25–30
Chicken breast, grilled	1 cup	25–30
Chicken meatballs and sliders (low fat)	3 meatballs or sliders	35
Chicken sausage (low fat, large)	2 links	25–30
Deli meat (roasted chicken breast)	4–5 oz.	25–30
Turkey		
Deli meat	4 oz.	25–30
Turkey breast, ground (99% fat free)	4 oz.	25–30
Turkey breast, skinless	4–5 oz.	25–30
Turkey burger (98% fat free)	1 burger	25–35
Pork		
Deli ham, extra lean	4–6 oz.	25–35
Pork chops, extra lean	4–6 oz.	25–35
Pork tenderloin, extra lean	4–6 oz.	25–35
Beef		
Beef, 98% lean	4–5 oz.	25–30
Beef, tenderloin	4–5 oz.	25–30
Beef, sirloin	4–5 oz.	25–30
Beef, top round	4–5 oz.	25–30
Deli meat, 97% lean	4 oz.	25–30
Veal, top round	4–5 oz.	25–30

	Serving	Protein (g)
Other		
Bison, steak medallions	1 steak	30–35
Lamb loin, lean	4–5 oz.	25–30
Venison	4–5 oz.	25–30
Seafood		
Bass	4–5 oz.	25–30
Bluefish	4–5 oz.	25–30
Catfish	4–5 oz.	25–30
Clams, canned in water	1 cup	25–30
Clams, fresh	20	25–30
Cod	4–5 oz.	25–30
Crab	4–5 oz.	25–30
Flounder	4–5 oz.	25–30
Grouper	4–5 oz.	25–30
Haddock	4–5 oz.	25–30
Halibut	4–5 oz.	25–30
Lobster	4–5 oz.	25–30
Mahi mahi	4–5 oz.	25–30
Orange roughy	4–5 oz.	25–30
Oyster	1 ¼ cup	25–30
Perch	4–5 oz.	25–30
Salmon	4–5 oz.	25–30
Salmon, canned, wild, Atlantic	½ cup	25–30
Sardines, in spring water, no salt added	5 oz.	25–30
Scallops	4–5 oz.	25–30
Sea bass	4–5 oz.	25–30

	Serving	Protein (g)
Seafood *(continued)*		
Shrimp	4–5 oz.	25–30
Snapper	4–5 oz.	25–30
Swordfish	4–5 oz.	25–30
Tilapia	4–5 oz.	25–30
Tuna, canned in water, white albacore	4–5 oz.	25–30
Tuna, yellow-fin	4–5 oz.	25–30
Turbot	4–5 oz.	25–30
Whitefish	4–5 oz.	25–30
Vegetarian *(see website for updated brand information)*		
Vegetarian soy breakfast links	4 links	16
Vegetarian soy burger such as tomato basil pizza burger	2 patties	22
Chicken-less strips	13 strips	30
Jumbo veggie links	2 links	30
Veggie breakfast patties	3 patties	30
Soy meatless tenders	1.5 tenders	30
Soy meatless burgers	3 patties	24
Beef-less ground beef-textured vegetable protein	1 cup	30
Edamame (blanched, shelled)	½ cup	13
Dry roasted edamame	¼ cup	14
Powdered peanut butter	4 tbsp.	10
Dairy		
1% cottage cheese	1 cup	28

Proteins for Combinations or Snacks

Proteins for Combinations or Snacks	Serving	Protein (g)
Meat		
Canadian bacon	2 slices	11
Turkey bacon	2 slices	12
Turkey sausage	4 links	10
Breakfast sausage (chicken and apple)	3 links	14
Chicken burgers (lean or low fat)	1 burger	22
Beef jerky	1 stick	8–10
Turkey pepperoni (low fat)	1 oz.	10
Chicken or turkey jerky	1 stick	12
Eggs		
Liquid egg substitute	½ cup	12
Egg combo (1 large egg plus 3 egg whites)	See item	17
Egg whites	5	17.5
Egg whites, liquid	½ cup	14
Eggs, whole	2 large	13
Hard-boiled egg whites	3 large	18
Milk and milk substitutes		
Almond milk (unsweetened vanilla flavor)	1 cup	1
Half and half, fat free	2 tbsp.	1
Soy milk, unsweetened	1 cup	7

	Serving	Protein (g)
Cheese		
Light Swiss cheese	1 oz.	8
Light cheese, in small rounds	2 rounds	12
Light cheddar cheese	1 oz.	8
Shredded cheese, 2% milk	1 oz.	8
Singles, fat free American	2 slices	8
Light cheese, triangles	4 wedges	10
Light ricotta cheese	½ cup	5
Light shredded cheese	1 oz.	8
Light or low-fat string cheese	2 sticks	12
Greek yogurt		
1% plain	6 oz.	18

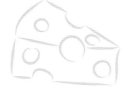

In addition, there are many preprepared protein foods on the market: protein shakes, protein soups, protein oatmeal, protein coffee drinks, hot chocolate. See the website for more information.

Vegetable Choices

Eat two cups of vegetables at lunch and two servings at dinner. If you prefer, you can also spread your vegetable servings out into different times during the day. It's perfectly fine to throw some onions or green peppers into your morning omelet. You will notice that, unlike the protein choices, there are no specific serving sizes listed. That is because I find it most unlikely that you will eat such an excessive amount of the vegetables on this list that it will impact your carbohydrate intake. Some people need more volume to feel full, and if that is the case, have more broccoli or cauliflower.

Vegetables

- Artichoke hearts
- Arugula
- Asparagus
- Bean sprouts
- Beets
- Broccoli
- Brussels sprouts
- Cabbage
- Carrots
- Cauliflower
- Celery
- Cucumber
- Eggplant
- Green beans
- Greens (collard, mustard, turnip)
- Leeks
- Lettuce (romaine or iceberg)
- Mushrooms
- Okra
- Onion
- Peppers (any color)
- Radishes
- Sauerkraut
- Shallots
- Snow peas
- Spaghetti squash
- Spinach
- Tomato
- Wax beans
- Zucchini

Ideal Salads

Make sure your salads contain 1–2 cups of lettuce, and you can add fresh low-carb vegetables like cucumbers, radishes, onions, and tomatoes to make them even more delicious.

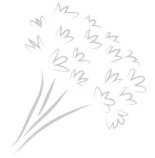

If you're not a lettuce lover:

- Try using shredded coleslaw mix

- Turn a large lettuce leaf into a wrap

- Thinly slice cucumbers and marinate them in rice vinegar.

For salad dressings, make sure the dressing you use contains no more than 5 grams of fat and 10 grams of carbs or less per 2 tablespoons. Use spritzer dressings, which coat and cover the salad nicely without using too much dressing.

Try these easy salad dressing ideas:

- 2–4 tablespoons of your favorite salsa

- Squeeze a lemon wedge with 1 tablespoon olive oil and a pinch of salt

- Rice vinegar with a pinch of ginger powder

The recipes in Part IV will give you many more enticing ideas.

If you dislike lettuce or if it doesn't agree with you, you can substitute more of the vegetables from the approved list. During the three reclaim days, do not add fruit, grains, or vegetables that are not on the list.

Beverages on the Reclaim Days

- Strive for 64 ounces of water each day.

- Have up to 2 cups of coffee, but do not add sugar. You can add up to a cup of unsweetened almond or soy milk from the dairy substitute list, as their carbohydrate content is low. You can add a splash of dairy milk, but avoid adding more than ⅛ cup due to the higher carbohydrate count. If fat-free half and half is desired, keep the serving to 2 tablespoons.

- Have up to 2 cups of black tea, with the same recommendations as above for coffee with regards to the addition of milk. Do not add sugar.

- You can also have green tea, hot or iced, or try herbal tea. Do not add sugar.

- Seltzer, as much as you like.

- As for calorie-free beverages with artificial sweeteners: you know my recommendations on this from Chapter 10, but if you cannot do without them, easing into changes is fine.

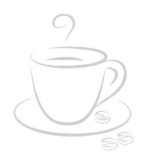

Reclaim Days Meal Plan Examples

Reclaim Day 1

Breakfast: 3 turkey sausage links, 1 cup cottage cheese 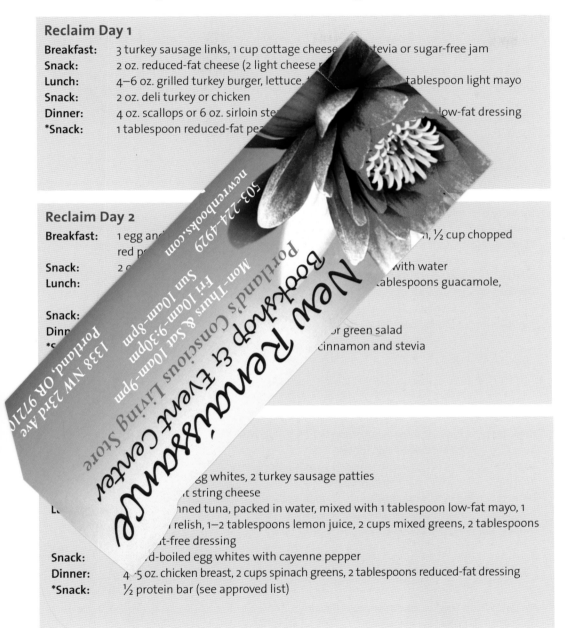 stevia or sugar-free jam
Snack: 2 oz. reduced-fat cheese (2 light cheese
Lunch: 4–6 oz. grilled turkey burger, lettuce, tablespoon light mayo
Snack: 2 oz. deli turkey or chicken
Dinner: 4 oz. scallops or 6 oz. sirloin stea low-fat dressing
*Snack: 1 tablespoon reduced-fat pea

Reclaim Day 2

Breakfast: 1 egg an ½ cup chopped
red pe
Snack: 2 o with water
Lunch: tablespoons guacamole,

Snack:
Dinner: or green salad
cinnamon and stevia

egg whites, 2 turkey sausage patties
t string cheese
nned tuna, packed in water, mixed with 1 tablespoon low-fat mayo, 1
relish, 1–2 tablespoons lemon juice, 2 cups mixed greens, 2 tablespoons
t-free dressing
Snack: d-boiled egg whites with cayenne pepper
Dinner: 4–5 oz. chicken breast, 2 cups spinach greens, 2 tablespoons reduced-fat dressing
*Snack: ½ protein bar (see approved list)

*Men should choose from the larger serving sizes. For example, if the meal suggestion calls for 4–5 oz., men should choose
5 oz. Additionally, men receive a third snack.

Reclaim Day 4

Breakfast: ½ cup plain Greek yogurt with sugar-free syrup, 3 slices Canadian bacon
Snack: 2 turkey deli rolls
Lunch: 5 oz. canned salmon in water, 2 cups of mixed greens, 2 tablespoons light dressing
Snack: ¼ cup dry roasted edamame
Dinner: 4–5 oz. chicken breast, 1 cup fresh green beans, ½ tomato, balsamic vinegar to taste
*Snack: 2 light cheese rounds

Reclaim Day 5

Breakfast: 1 ¼ cups liquid egg whites, 1 oz. light shredded cheese
Snack: 2 oz. lean deli meat
Lunch: 2 vegetarian soy burgers (see website for recommendations), 1 slice reduced-fat cheese, 1–2 cups mixed greens, 2 tablespoons light dressing
Snack: ½ cup reduced-fat cottage cheese with sliced tomato
Dinner: 4–5 oz. grouper, 1 cup mixed greens, 2 tablespoons light dressing, 1 cup roasted zucchini
*Snack: 2 tablespoons light cream cheese and vegetables

Reclaim Day 6

Breakfast: 2 vegetarian soy sausage patties, ½ cup liquid egg whites
Snack: 3 hard-boiled egg whites
Lunch: 4–5 oz. grilled shrimp, 1–2 cups mixed greens, 2 tablespoons light dressing
Snack: 2 pieces light string cheese
Dinner: 4–5 oz. pork tenderloin, 1 cup mixed greens, 2 tablespoons light dressing, 1 cup steamed broccoli/cauliflower
*Snack: 1 tablespoon peanut butter with celery

*Men should choose from the larger serving sizes. For example if the meal suggestion calls for 4–5 oz., men should choose 5 oz. Additionally, men receive a third snack.

Transformation

Congratulations! You have completed the Reclaim Days. You are now ready to proceed with the Transformation days.

Transformation days are designed to keep your energy level high, your appetite satisfied, and your body locked into a fat-burning mode. As you can see from the weight loss calendar, the majority of your days are spent in this cycle until you reach the new you, which is lifelong health and well-being.

The most important concept during Transformation days is that you still must get 25–35 grams of protein with each meal and 10–20 grams of protein with each snack and that your carbohydrate amount at each meal and over the course of the entire day must be balanced to keep the **MD Factor** symptoms away. This will allow you to lose weight without being hungry, nip cravings in the bud, and keep you energized all day.

The way you'll be eating is:

- Choose protein five to six times per day

- Choose vegetables four times per day

- Green salads with fresh vegetables two times per day

- Choose fruit or healthful carbohydrates from the list no more than two times per day

In other words, you'll be eating a lot of protein, including meat, poultry, eggs, and fish; a large variety of vegetables; and some fruit and fats, both of which will add sweetness and flavor to your diet. You'll be limiting carbohydrates by initially cutting out white bread, white potatoes, pasta (even whole-grain pasta), rice (even brown rice), chocolate, baked goods, sugary desserts, and sweets.

The most important piece of the weight loss puzzle is protein.

The Transformation Key

- You need to eat sufficient protein at every meal (25–35 grams) and watch your carbohydrates so the daily total is 100 grams or less per day.

- Eat meals and snacks every two to three hours. Don't skip any meals or snacks during the day!

Protein Is Paramount

It bears repeating: the most important piece of the weight loss puzzle is protein. Without the basis of lean protein to make up the majority of your meals, your metabolism will not begin to regroup and retrain your system to burn fat. The ideal serving of protein is 25–35 grams at every meal. This meets the protein threshold you need so that your body can begin absorbing all the amino acids it needs, which helps regulate insulin. It is crucial to hit that 25–35 gram mark at every meal. If you fall short, you may be a lot hungrier, and your body will resist weight loss. Toward that end, please pay careful attention to the serving sizes I've listed on the protein choices for the Transformation days. Yes, if you choose cottage cheese, I want you to have 1 cup of cottage cheese, not the ¼ or ½ cup that's listed as the serving size on the container" You need to get as close as you can to 25–35 grams at each meal.

Just like in the Reclaim phase, in the Transformation phase there are two ways to get the amount of protein I suggest for each meal. First, you can choose one of the protein foods I've listed here—the serving sizes will give you that necessary 25–35 grams. You can also choose to combine protein foods to give you some variety while still ensuring that you get the right amount of protein. For example, you could have 1¼ cups of liquid egg whites, which will give you 30 grams of protein, or you could have ½ cup of liquid egg whites (which provides 12 grams of protein) plus 2 slices of turkey bacon (for another 12 grams of protein) and then 1 cup of skim milk, 1% milk, or soy milk (which has 7–8 grams of protein). With that combination you are at 32 grams of protein.

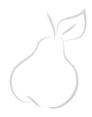

Transformation Carbohydrates

Certain foods encourage your pancreas to release a huge amount of insulin. You know what the culprits are—the kind of foods that are full of sugar and fat and empty carbs and are very hard to stop eating! But you also know that when you have the **MD Factor**, your metabolic signals get all mixed up, and any excess sugar that comes from these carbs will be stored as fat.

You can easily stop this mix-up from happening at all if you eat less than 100 grams of carbohydrates per day. Your body will not release much insulin when carb levels are that low.

Please note: Your carbohydrates need to be spread over the day, just as your proteins are. If you eat all 100 grams of your carbohydrate allotment at one sitting, you will have a large release of insulin to handle all those carbs. This big surge of insulin will probably be followed by a blood sugar dip that will both induce and increase your appetite. We don't want appetite stimulation, so spread out your healthful carbs and stick to the portion sizes given for the fruits, starches, and grains.

Understand How to Count Net Carbs

All carbohydrates are not created equal. Many foods are called carbohydrates, but the only ones you need to limit are the carbs that trigger your **MD Factor** and raise your blood sugar.

For example, sugar alcohols such as maltitol, sorbitol, and erythritol are added to foods to create a sweet flavor, and they'll be listed on food labels as carbs—but they don't raise your blood sugar when you eat them.

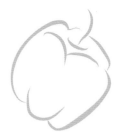

Nor does fiber. This includes dietary fiber, which is sometimes listed as soluble or insoluble fiber. Soluble fiber, found in fruits such as apples and in beans, is digestible and can help remove cholesterol from your bloodstream. Insoluble fiber is found in green leafy vegetables and is not digestible. It gives bulk and roughage and helps move food through your digestive system.

For more information about the exact amount of carbohydrate in various foods and to learn how to calculate net carbs, please see Appendix C. You will not exceed the carbohydrate recommendation of 100 grams per day necessary for the Transformation phase if you eat the recommended serving sizes listed for fruits and healthful carbohydrates. You can still eat as much of the vegetables and salads on the approved list as you want.

Appendix F contains a more complete list of the carbohydrate counts in food. If you are a numbers person, you may want to track your total for each meal and the day. This may also help you if you have a very stubborn **MD Factor,** as keeping a closer tab on the carb total will make a difference in your weight loss.

Snacks

Just like during the Reclaim days, during the Transformation days it is absolutely essential that you eat every two to three hours in order to keep the **MD Factor** at bay and your blood sugar levels stable. Snacks containing between 10 and 20 grams of protein are the best way to combat the **MD Factor**.

If you miss a snack, make sure you eat it later, or else it will be a challenge to meet your daily protein goal.

Transformation Days for Women

Breakfast: 25–30 g protein, 1 serving healthful carbs from the approved list, vitamin and mineral supplement, 16 oz. water

Snack: 10–15 g protein from snack list, 8 oz. water

Lunch: 25–30 g protein, 1 serving healthful carbs from the approved list, 1–2 cups cooked or raw vegetables from approved list, 1–2 cups salad, 16 oz. water

Snack: 10–15 g protein from the approved list, 8 oz. water

Dinner: 25–30 g protein, 1–2 cups cooked or raw vegetables, 1–2 cups salad, 16 oz. water

Transformation Days for Men

Breakfast: 25–35 g protein, 1 serving healthful carbs from the approved list, vitamin and mineral supplement, 16 oz. water

Snack: 10–20 g protein from snack list, 8 oz. water

Lunch: 25–35 g protein, 1 serving healthful carbs from the approved list, 1–2 cups cooked or raw vegetables from approved list, 1–2 cups salad, 16 oz. water

Snack: 10–20 g protein from the approved list, 8 oz. water

Dinner: 25–35 g protein, 1–2 cups cooked or raw vegetables, 1–2 cups salad, 16 oz. water

*Snack: 10–20 g protein from the approved list

*Men should choose from the larger serving sizes. For example if the meal suggestion calls for 4–5 oz., men should choose 5 oz. Additionally, men receive a third snack.

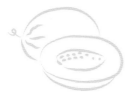

Healthy Complex Carbohydrates

Beans and Grains

Black beans	½ cup cooked
Black-eyed peas	½ cup cooked
Lentils	½ cup
Quinoa	½ cup
Garbanzo beans	½ cup cooked
Hummus	¼ cup
Red beans	½ cup cooked
Kidney beans	½ cup cooked
Brown rice	½ cup

Fruits

Apple	1 baseball-size	Mango	½ cup, diced
Apricots	4 halves, dried	Nectarine	1 medium
Banana	½ medium size	Orange	1 small
Blackberries	⅔ cup	Papaya	½ cup, cubed
Blueberries	⅔ cup	Peach	1 baseball-size
Cantaloupe	1 cup	Pear	½ light-bulb-size
Cherries	10 grape-size	Persimmon	1 medium size
Dates	2 dried	Pineapple	½ cup, cubed
Grapefruit	½ fruit	Plum	1 medium
Grapes	15 small	Raspberries	⅔ cup
Honeydew	⅛ melon	Strawberries	1 cup, sliced
Kiwi	1 medium size	Tangerine	1 medium size
Mandarin orange	1 tennis-ball-size	Watermelon	1 cup, cubed

Beverages on Transformation Days

- Strive for 64 ounces of water each day.

- Have up to 2 cups of coffee, but continue to avoid sugar. Dairy, soy, or almond milk are okay.

- Have up to 2 cups of black tea. Dairy, soy, or almond milk are okay. Continue to avoid sugar.

- You can also have green tea, hot or iced, or try herbal tea. Do not add sugar.

- Seltzer, as much as you like.

- As for calorie-free beverages with artificial sweeteners: you know my recommendations on this from Chapter 10, but if you cannot do without them, easing into changes is fine.

Transformation Days Meal Plan Examples

Your goals are 120–140 grams of protein, 60–100 grams of carbohydrates, and less than 40 grams of fat.

Transformation Day 1

Breakfast: 2 eggs scrambled, 2 turkey sausage links, 2/3 cup blueberries

Snack: 5 oz. plain or vanilla low-fat or non-fat Greek yogurt

Lunch: 5 oz. canned tuna, mixed with 1 tablespoon of light mayo, served over lettuce and tomato, with a side of tomato tabbouleh salad (see page 203)

Snack: ¼ cup walnuts, almonds, or pecans (limit to 2 times per week)

Dinner: Spaghetti squash with chicken and vegetable stuffing with green bean and tomato salad (see page 195)

*Snack: 2–3 slices of lean low-sodium deli meat, wrap around a dill pickle

Transformation Day 2

Breakfast: 1 cup low-fat or fat-free cottage cheese, 1 cup strawberries

Snack: 1 oz., about 1 slice, of smoked salmon rolled with 1–2 tablespoons reduced-fat cream cheese

Lunch: 4–5 oz. grilled chicken with French Lentil Salad (page 204)

Snack: 1 oz. reduced-fat cheese, 7 slices turkey pepperoni

Dinner: Halibut and spinach (see page 189) with Cauliflower Rice (see page 202)

*Snack: Edamole High-Protein Guacamole (see page 211)

*Men should choose from the larger serving sizes. For example, if the meal suggestion calls for 4–5 oz., men should choose 5 oz. Additionally, men receive a third snack.

Transformation Day 3

Breakfast: Broccoli and cheese omelet (½ cup egg whites, ¼ cup cooked broccoli, ¼ cup low-fat shredded cheese, salt and pepper to taste), served with 1 cup cubed cantaloupe

Snack: 10–15 grams of whey or rice protein powder with 8 oz. water/skim milk or unsweetened rice/almond milk, add cinnamon or fresh nutmeg

Lunch: Stir fry made with 1 cup fresh or frozen mixed vegetables, 4 oz. shrimp or chicken, served over ¼ cup brown rice or quinoa

Snack: 2 light string cheese sticks

Dinner: Eggplant Rollatini (see page 198) with side of arugula salad, add several cherry tomatoes, mushrooms, and 1 oz. shaved Parmesan cheese, 1–2 teaspoons olive oil, 1–2 teaspoons fresh squeezed lemon juice, salt and pepper to taste

*Snack: One serving of high protein breakfast cereal dry or with skim milk or unsweetened almond milk

Transformation Day 4

Breakfast: Oatmeal cottage cheese pancakes: combine ¼ cup oatmeal, ¼ cup low-fat or non-fat cottage cheese, ½ teaspoon vanilla, 2 egg whites in a blender. Spray skillet with cooking spray, and cook batter in silver dollar sizes. Serve with 3 slices of Canadian bacon

Snack: ½ cup skim milk ricotta cheese, choose either cinnamon or cocoa power to taste, add Stevia, ¼ cup canned pumpkin, and 1 teaspoon pumpkin pie spice

Lunch: Chef Salad with 1.5 oz. ham, 1.5 oz. turkey, 1 oz. low-fat cheese, 1 hard-boiled egg white, ½ cup cucumber, ½ cup carrots, ½ cup sliced red bell pepper, ½ cup tomatoes, thinly sliced red onion, 2 cups romaine lettuce, 1–2 tablespoons light dressing, plus a side of one serving of fruit

Snack: 1.5 oz. turkey, chicken, salmon, or bison jerky

Dinner: Chicken Cacciatore with Italian Green Beans (see page 193)

*Snack 1–2 tablespoons of peanut butter or almond butter with celery

Transformation Day 5

Breakfast: Pumpkin Delight Smoothie: 2 scoops of vanilla whey or rice protein powder, ½ cup canned organic pumpkin, 1 teaspoon pumpkin pie spice, vanilla extract, 8–12 oz. of water or unsweetened almond milk blended

Snack: ½ cup fat-free or low-fat cottage cheese sprinkled with cinnamon

Lunch: English muffin pizza made on a light English muffin, tomato paste, oregano, ½ cup light shredded mozzarella cheese, 2–3 oz. of shredded chicken or turkey pepperoni, peppers, and mushrooms. Add an Italian salad of lettuce, tomato, cucumber, mushrooms, and 3 olives with light balsamic vinaigrette

Snack: 1–2 tablespoons of hummus with chips made from thinly sliced cucumbers, squash, or zucchini

Dinner: Turkey Burgers and Slaw (see page 188) with slices of fresh cucumbers and tomatoes

*Snack: 3 hard-boiled egg whites with salt, pepper, and paprika

Transformation Day 6

Breakfast: Mexican Omelet (½ cup egg whites, ¼ cup red and green peppers, ¼ cup mushrooms, ½ cup onion, ½ oz. shredded Mexican cheese), topped with ¼ cup salsa

Snack: Lightly salted edamame, choose from 1 cup in pods, ½ cup shelled, or ¼ cup dry roasted

Lunch: 3 oz. turkey breast, low-carb pita, lettuce, tomato, mustard, and dill pickles with a Greek salad of tomato, red onion, 3 Kalamata olives, and ½–1 oz. feta cheese crumbles

Snack: 2 reduced-fat cheese rounds

Dinner: Lemon and Rosemary Chicken with Turkey Bacon Brussels Sprouts (see page 194)

*Snack ¼ cup lightly salted sunflower or pumpkin seeds

*Men should choose from the larger serving sizes. For example, if the meal suggestion calls for 4–5 oz., men should choose 5 oz. Additionally, men receive a third snack.

CHAPTER 12

Keeping Track of Your Progress

When my patients start working with me on their **MD Factor** Action Plan, they follow up with their dietitian to assess their progress, have any questions answered, get more ideas for meal plans, and also to help with accountability. Think of this chapter as your own personal session, as I'm including all the information shared one-on-one with patients. Take the Well-Being & Metabolism Correction Quiz located on page 17, write down your answers, and recheck yourself every week to track the improvement in your well-being and metabolism.

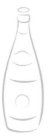

Week 1 Check-In

Checklist

Place a check mark next to each of the things you accomplished this week.

❑ I wrote down all the food I consumed each day in my log

❑ I followed the 25–35 gram protein rule and chose my carbs from the approved lists

❑ I ate my snacks each day

❑ I ate every two to three hours

❑ I took my multivitamin each day

❑ I drank at least eight glasses or four 16-oz. bottles of water

❑ I did not feel hungry this week

❑ I slept well this week

❑ I had energy this week

❑ I had regular bowel movements this week

❑ I lost weight after seven days of following the meal plan

❑ I lost _____ pounds since I began following the meal plan

If you did not accomplish every item on the checklist, don't get discouraged. Mastering the **MD Factor** Action Plan is a new skill, and all new skills take time to learn and do. If you got derailed, or if someone convinced you to order dessert, don't beat yourself up. Make a new agreement and commitment and move forward.

Week 2 Check-In

By now you should have far fewer cravings for sugar and the carbs you used to eat, as well as a more stable energy level throughout the day. You may be noticing that you're sleeping better, with a lot less fatigue in the afternoon when you used to want to nap. Most people also feel more level, with a satisfying mental clarity.

Most important, you should have noticed that you have lost weight— anywhere between four and ten pounds is normal.

If you haven't lost weight yet, review what you've been eating and see if there is anything you can change to make it more like the meal plans in this book, which are proven to work. If you are eating less or skipping snacks, you are likely slowing your metabolic rate, and this can definitely slow your weight loss.

If you are not moving your bowels regularly, this can also slow weight loss significantly. I recommend that you take a fiber supplement, such as any product with psyllium husk or other powdered fiber you mix in water, as well as a magnesium supplement, which you read about in Chapter 7. Also ensure you are drinking at least 64 ounces of water every day.

At this point, I recommend strapping on a pedometer and beginning to record the number of steps you take each day. As you know, I don't recommend throwing yourself into a full-bore exercise plan right away when you start the program, but becoming aware of how much you move each day is really helpful.

Studies show that getting fewer than five thousand steps a day is associated with being overweight. Your goal is to move up to ten thousand steps or more each day. You can easily add to your total steps by parking your car farther away in the lot from your destination, taking stairs, and going for short walks.

During the Transformation phase, it's best to get on the scale in the morning no more than once per week. Record your weight and compare it to the previous week's weight. A weigh-in every day can be misleading, because your body will always have natural fluctuations from water, fat, and gas. Some people get incredibly discouraged if they don't lose weight every day, but they still may be losing fat and showing no movement due simply to water retention. These weight fluctuations are very common when you start the **MD Factor** Action Plan.

I urge you to stick to the **MD Factor** Action Plan meal plan long enough to see your body fat change—I have many years of clinical data showing how well it works. You will have significant fat loss while lean muscle mass is maintained. Don't give up even before you really started because the scale seems so stubborn! A much better way to measure your progress is when your clothes suddenly feel loose and your waistline is smaller. If you follow the meal plan closely, you will lose body fat and that is your ultimate goal.

What Should I Do If I Get Off Track?

If you get off track—perhaps you were traveling on business, had important family events, had a cold, or just needed a break—restarting the Reclaim days for up to three days maximum is the perfect way to regroup. They are also very helpful if you find sugar cravings beginning to creep back in. It is also helpful to download a meal plan template from the website, **www.MDFactorBook.com**, and start tracking your carbs as well as protein. You may find that you have inadvertently had more than 100 grams on some days.

Week 3 Check-In

Free Meals

An important part of the **MD Factor** Action Plan is a Free Meal or "My Night." This is one meal, once each week, where you can indulge! Have a dessert, or go for that popcorn at a movie.

Your Free Meal is a great way to help you avoid feeling deprived, or as if you are always "on a diet." The key is to follow up a Free Meal by restarting your next meal with a Transformation meal. It's a great way to get back to your metabolism-correcting meal plan.

Start your Free Meals after three weeks on the **MD Factor** Action Plan. By then, you should be in a groove with your meals and snacks, and your **MD Factor** should be going away.

Some patients, however, are afraid that adding a Free Meal or even one "cheat" food will trigger cravings and send them back to old habits. If you feel this way, wait a few more weeks or even a month or two and then try it. By then, your **MD Factor** should be under control, and eating a higher-carbohydrate meal won't trigger large blood sugar fluctuations.

Free Snacks on Transformation Days

If you've had a sweet tooth for many years and are struggling with needing a sweet flavor or a satisfying substitute for your favorite dessert, try adding one of these low-cal, low-sugar cookie, pudding, ice pop, or ice cream choices to your meal plan. This does not take the place of any meal or snack, so please be sure you eat this in addition to your recommended meals. Check **www.MDFactorBook.com** for updated lists of these low-sugar treats.

Week 4 Check-In

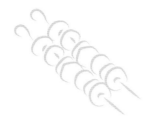

After nearly a month, you should be feeling a lot better, with improved energy, mood, sleeping habits, stamina, and mental clarity. Your weight is steadily coming off, your cravings are way down, and you're thrilled.

But this is also the point in the **MD Factor** Action Plan where the honeymoon often begins to end.

This is the ideal time to make your meals and snacks even more interesting. Don't stick with the meals you've been eating so faithfully, unless you find it easier that way. Keep it fun! My patients see my dietitians every week in part to keep it fresh. They share lots of incredibly yummy recipes and different flavor combinations.

Now is the time to use the recipes in Part IV. They've been tested by my experienced team of dieticians and chefs, so you get maximum weight loss as well as an incredible range of deliciousness.

For continually updated recipes and food combinations, please visit **www.MDFactorBook.com**.

BistroMD: Delivers the **MD Factor** Diet Directly to Your Door

Over my many years of fine-tuning, I know that the meal plans work. My patients feel better within a week or two, and their intense cravings for sugar and junk food carbs have significantly decreased. They've learned to enjoy eating real food in appropriate portion sizes without ever feeling starved or deprived.

The only negative comment I sometimes receive is that eating this way takes a lot of planning and a lot of work. Especially for those who aren't used to cooking!

This comment is valid, because eating well does take more time than many of us have. I know how hard it can be to shop for, prepare, and cook meals around specific parameters when you are strapped for time. (There's a reason fast-food restaurants are so popular, and the time factor is a big part of it.) I've always been incredibly busy with my education, a demanding career, and a family with four children, so I share the crazy schedule many of my patients have. We've all got work, homework help, the endless pickups and drop-offs at sports and school events and play dates, shopping, housework, maybe trying to see our spouses once in a while, and trying to fit in time to exercise and have a moment to ourselves. I'm sure you know the feeling!

I must also confess that I've never enjoyed cooking or meal preparation, especially if it involves trimming or cooking meat. I never manage to time everything so all the components of the meal come out at the same time. I was like so many of my patients and ate primarily for convenience until about seventeen years ago, when my husband and I tucked our toddlers (who are now teenagers) into bed one night, hurried into the kitchen, and then polished off an entire pizza. We looked at each other, and that was it.

"We are killing ourselves," we said, and we knew we had to make some real changes.

So, yes, there are many days when it would be so much easier for me to just eat a bowl of cereal and then graze on fruit or crackers, or eat out. But these are exactly all the things I know trigger the **MD Factor** and put me at risk for future medical problems.

I don't want my patients to fall into a rut of chicken and broccoli with a salad every night, because creating sauces and side dishes with low carb counts takes time. It's worth it to have the meal be special—but that won't work if you can't find the time to concoct such meals!

To tackle this situation, I created bistroMD several years ago. I brought the protein, carbohydrate, and fat requirements for each meal and snack to several chefs and asked them to create meals that would not only fit the nutritional numbers but also taste sensational. I was thrilled to be able to create a program that unchains the user from the pressure and stress of eating healthy while still providing all of the benefits of correcting metabolism dysfunction. I eat these meals for my lunches and dinners many nights of the week to help me maintain my weight in a healthy range.

BistroMD is a labor of love, as the meals are created with high-quality ingredients without nitrates, phosphates, other chemicals or additives, or even the ridiculously and dangerously high sodium levels frequently found in frozen or other convenience meals. My philosophy has been that if I won't eat it or feel good about feeding it to my children or my patients, there is no way it will be allowed onto the bistroMD menu!

*The bistroMD diet delivery program differs slightly from the **MD Factor** Action Plan outlined in this book. To learn more, see Appendix H on page 239.*

For more information, go to **www.MDFactorBook.com**.

CHAPTER 13

The MD Factor Maintenance Plan

After you've been following the **MD Factor** Action Plan for four weeks, you move on to the Stabilization Phase. This is designed to prevent your body from getting too used to eating fewer calories than normal and slowing down your metabolic rate. When this happens, even if you are following the **MD Factor** Action Plan perfectly, your weight can plateau. This is one of the reasons people on low-calorie diets get frustrated and quit.

There is an easy way to prevent this, and that's precisely what the Stabilization phase will do over a two-week cycle.

✔ During each Stabilization Day, eat two to three more servings of healthful carbohydrates.

✔ Add these carbs into your meals.

✔ You should be eating between four and five servings of healthful carbs on these days.

Stabilization Phase Schedule

6 STABILIZATION DAYS
Women: 120 grams of protein, 100–150 grams of net carbs, 30–40 grams of fat
Men: 140 grams of protein, 100–150 grams of net carbs, 40–60 grams of fat

1 RECLAIM DAY
Women: 120 grams of protein, less than 60 grams of net carbs, 30 grams of fat
Men: 140 grams of protein, less than 60 grams of net carbs, 40 grams of fat

6 STABILIZATION DAYS

1 RECLAIM DAY

RESUME YOUR TRANSFORMATION DAYS
Women: 120 grams of protein, 60–100 grams of net carbs, 30 grams of fat
Men: 140 grams of protein, 60–100 grams of net carbs, 40 grams of fat

Continue this cycle until you reach your goal weight. Then move on to the Maintenance Phase.

Most of my patients continue to lose weight during the Stabilization phase. If, however, you follow the Stabilization phase and gain more than 1½ pounds per week, you may have a stubborn **MD Factor**. Wait another cycle or two before trying it again; sometimes it takes a few cycles for your body to adjust. If it doesn't, read about the supplements helpful to defeat the **MD Factor** in Chapter 7. Also look at the information about the medication metformin and discuss that with your physician, as you might need an extra boost to help reverse the **MD Factor**.

Stabilization Days

Stabilization Days for Women

Breakfast: 25–30 g protein, 1 serving healthful carbs from the approved list, vitamin and mineral supplement, 16 oz. water

Snack: 10–15 g protein, 8 oz. water, option of healthful carb serving

Lunch: 25–30 g protein, 1 serving healthful carbs from the approved list, 1–2 cups cooked or raw vegetables, 1–2 cups salad, 16 oz. water

Snack: 10–15 g protein, 8 oz. water

Dinner: 25–30 g protein, 1 serving healthful carbs from the approved list, 1–2 cups cooked or raw vegetables, 1–2 cups salad, 16 oz. water

Stabilization Days for Men

Breakfast: 25–35 g protein, 1 serving healthful carbs from the approved list, vitamin and mineral supplement, 16 oz. water

Snack: 10–20 g protein, 8 oz. water, option of healthful carb serving

Lunch: 25–35 g protein, 1 serving healthful carbs from the approved list, 1–2 cups cooked or raw vegetables, 1–2 cups salad, 16 oz. water

Snack: 10–20 g protein, 8 oz. water

Dinner: 25–35 g protein, 1 serving healthful carbs from the approved list, 1–2 cups cooked or raw vegetables, 1–2 cups salad, 16 oz. water

Snack: 10–20 g protein, option of healthful carb serving

Stabilization Phase: Additional Food to Eat

	Serving	Protein	Net carbs	Fat	Fiber
Cereals and Breads					
High fiber cereals*	½ – ¾ cup	2–4	8–18	1–1.5	10–14
Protein-supplemented cereal*	½ – ¾ cup	10	9	3	5
100% whole-wheat bread	1 slice	3–4	8–10	1	2
Whole-wheat English muffin	½ muffin	3	11	0.5	2
1 low-carb wrap	1 wrap	9	8	2.5	9
1 low-carb pita	1 pita	6	4	2	4

STARCHES	Serving	Protein	Net carbs	Fat	Fiber
Whole-Grain and Starchy Carbs					
Whole-wheat macaroni, cooked	½ cup	4	16.5	0.5	2
Whole-wheat spaghetti, cooked	½ cup	4	15.5	0.5	3
Couscous, cooked	½ cup	3.5	20	Trace	1.5
Brown rice, cooked	½ cup	2	21.5	0.5	1.5
Wild rice, cooked	½ cup	3	17	Trace	0.75
Baked Potato with skin	3 oz.	1.5	20.5	0	1.5
Baked sweet potato with skin	3 oz.	1.5	18.5	0	2.5
Mashed potatoes	½ cup	2	15.5	4	2
Oat bran bagel	½ bagel	4	18	1	1
Whole-wheat pita, 6-inch diameter	½ pita	3	15	1	2.5
Whole-wheat tortilla	1 tortilla	4	24	2.5	2
Whole-wheat roll	1 small	2.5	12.5	1	2
Whole-wheat bread	1 slice	4	10	1	2
Corn	½ cup	2	13.5	1	1.5
Quinoa	½ cup	5.5	27	2.5	2.5
Oatmeal (uncooked)	¼ cup	3	11.5	1.3	2

*Check the website www.MDFactorBook.com for brands and updated nutritional information.

The MD Factor Diet

Stabilization Days Meal Plan Examples

Your goals are 120 grams of protein, 100–150 grams of net carbohydrates, and less than 40–60 grams of fat.

Stabilization Day 1

Breakfast: 1 whole-wheat English muffin, 2 egg whites (or ½ cup of liquid egg substitute), 1 slice low-fat cheese, 1 slice lean Canadian bacon

Snack: sliced apple, 2 oz. light cheese

Lunch: 1 slice whole-wheat bread, 3–5 oz. deli ham, 1 oz. cheese placed in toaster for an open face melt, deli pickle, fresh carrots and cucumber

Snack: protein bar with 10 g protein, low carb

Dinner: 3–5 oz. shredded chicken with cup salsa, ½ cup black beans, 1 tablespoon low-fat sour cream, ¼ cup reduced-fat Mexican cheese, bed of lettuce

*Snack: 3 hard-boiled egg whites with a little salt and pepper, 20 grapes

Stabilization Day 2

Breakfast: ½ cup oatmeal, 3 pieces Canadian bacon, 2 hard-boiled egg whites

Snack: 1.5 oz. beef jerky

Lunch: 1 low-carb wrap, 3–5 oz. chicken, ¼ cup Parmesan cheese, 1 cup chopped lettuce or baby spinach leaves, 1 tablespoon low-fat Caesar dressing, ¼ cup hummus with carrots or celery

Snack: 7–8 wheat thins or nut thins with 2 tablespoons light cream cheese

Dinner: ½ cup whole-wheat pasta with ¼ cup red sauce (measure the pasta carefully), 5–10 large shrimp sautéed in 1 tablespoon light olive oil with ½ cup zucchini, ½ cup yellow squash, and ¼ cup chopped onion

*Snack: 1 light yogurt

Stabilization Day 3

Breakfast: Breakfast Frittata (see page 197), 2 slices turkey bacon, 2 slices whole-wheat toast, 1 tablespoon light or sugar-free jelly

Snack: ½ cup 1% plain Greek yogurt with ⅔ cup blackberries

Lunch: Curry Chicken Salad (see page 199) over 1–2 cups greens, 1 toasted low-carb pita, 15 grapes

Snack: ¼ cup dry roasted edamame

Dinner: 4–5 oz. salmon served with Pepper Coulis (see page 209), ¼ cup cooked quinoa blended with chopped spinach and olives

*Snack: 1 oz. lean deli meat, 1 oz. reduced-fat cheese, 3 **MD Factor** approved crackers

*Men should choose from the larger serving sizes. For example, if the meal suggestion calls for 4–5 oz., men should choose 5 oz. Additionally, men receive a third snack.

Stabilization Day 4

Breakfast:	2 veggie sausage patties, 2 eggs (or ½ cup egg substitute), ⅔ cup raspberries
Snack:	½ cup 1% cottage cheese, ½ cup diced pineapple
Lunch:	Grilled Mediterranean Kabobs (see page 197), 1 low-carb wrap, 1 cup Dill Cucumber Salad (see page 201)
Snack:	1 stick beef jerky, ¼ cup hummus with raw vegetables
Dinner:	Lemon Chicken Picatta with Squash Ribbons (see page 190), 1 small whole-wheat roll, 1 cup spinach salad with 2 dried apricots
*Snack:	1 tablespoon peanut butter with celery stalks

Stabilization Day 5

Breakfast:	¾ cup high fiber cereal with ½ medium banana, ½ cup skim milk. 1 cup liquid egg whites blended with ½ cup vegetables (see page 150), 1 oz. light shredded cheese
Snack:	¼ cup nuts, 1 cup strawberries
Lunch:	4–5 oz. chicken breast with Garlic Velouté (see page 208), ½ cup French Lentil Salad (see page 204), 1–2 cups of fresh greens. Combine all ingredients.
Snack:	2 light cheese rounds, 1 small apple
Dinner:	Pork chops with onion-mushroom gravy and Cauliflower Mash (see page 191), 1 cup roasted Brussels sprouts, ½ cup cooked wild rice
*Snack:	½ protein bar from **MD Factor** approved list

Stabilization Day 6

Breakfast:	2 slices turkey bacon, egg combo (1 large egg + 3 egg whites), 1 cup cantaloupe
Snack:	2 tablespoons light cream cheese on vegetables
Lunch:	4–5 oz. turkey burger, 1 slice reduced-fat swiss cheese, ¼ cup Mango Salsa (see page 207) for burger topping, 1 whole-wheat bun, 1 cup fresh salad greens with ¼ mango salsa
Snack:	1 cup light ricotta cheese mixed with cinnamon, 1 medium sliced peach
Dinner:	Old-Fashioned Beef Stew (see page 196), 1 small baked potato with skin, 1–2 cups fresh salad greens
*Snack:	1 tablespoon hummus, 1 oz. deli meat

*Men should choose from the larger serving sizes. For example, if the meal suggestion calls for 4–5 oz., men should choose 5 oz. Additionally, men receive a third snack.

Moving from the Stabilization Phase to the Maintenance Phase

Stabilization days form the backbone of your Maintenance Phase. Eating the right amount of lean protein every day will keep the weight off, and most people are able to reintroduce healthful portions of carbohydrates and fats spread throughout the day and not gain weight.

Follow these guidelines:

- The best way to add these important additional calories is by slowly increasing your servings of fruit, vegetables, beans, and some whole grains.

- Nuts are a healthful snack, containing protein and healthful fat.

- Occasional treats such as desserts, chocolate, and wine are important to add—but remember, most people can't eat dessert every day and keep the pounds off.

- You might want to weigh yourself daily instead of weekly, as your weight shouldn't be fluctuating very much at this point.

- If a few pounds are starting to creep back, you have added too much to your plan, or you might still have the **MD Factor**. Restart your three Reclaim days. Then go back on Transformation for two more weeks until your weight is where you want it to be.

- Make sure to exercise!

The **MD Factor** Action Plan Schedule

3 RECLAIM DAYS

25 TRANSFORMATION DAYS

6 STABILIZATION DAYS

1 RECLAIM DAY

6 STABILIZATION DAYS

1 RECLAIM DAY

Repeat the Metabolism-Correcting Meal Plan Rotation

28 TRANSFORMATION DAYS

6 STABILIZATION DAYS

1 RECLAIM DAY

6 STABILIZATION DAYS

1 RECLAIM DAY

Your Maintenance Calendar

The easiest way to keep track of your **MD Factor** Action Plan schedule is with a calendar. Use this template to help you with your schedule.

Monday	Tuesday	Wednesday	Thursday	Friday	Saturday	Sunday
Day 1 R	Day 2 R	Day 3 R	Day 4 T	Day 5 T	Day 6 T	Day 7 T
Day 8 T	Day 9 T	Day 10 T	Day 11 T	Day 12 T	Day 13 T	Day 14 T
Day 15 T	Day 16 T	Day 17 T	Day 18 T	Day 19 * T	Day 20 T	Day 21 T
Day 22 T	Day 23 T	Day 24 T	Day 25 T	Day 26 * T	Day 27 T	Day 28 T
Day 29 S	Day 30 S	Day 31 S	Day 32 S	Day 33 * S	Day 34 S	Day 35 R
Day 36 S	Day 37 S	Day 38 S	Day 39 S	Day 40 * S	Day 41 S	Day 42 R
Day 43 T	Day 44 T	Day 45 T	Day 46 T	Day 47 * T	Day 48 T	Day 49 T
Day 50 T	Day 51 T	Day 52 T	Day 53 T	Day 54 * T	Day 55 T	Day 56 T
Day 57 T	Day 58 T	Day 59 T	Day 60 T	Day 61 * T	Day 62 T	Day 63 T
Day 64 T	Day 65 T	Day 66 T	Day 67 T	Day 68 * T	Day 69 T	Day 70 T
Day 71 S	Day 72 S	Day 73 S	Day 74 S	Day 75 * S	Day 76 S	Day 77 R
Day 78 S	Day 79 S	Day 80 S	Day 81 S	Day 82 * S	Day 83 S	Day 84 R

R = Reclaim days, for insulin sensitizing: less than 60 grams of net carbs
S = Stabilization days: between 100 and 150 grams of net carbs
T = Transformation days, for weight loss: between 60 and 100 grams of net carbs
*Represents a structured break from the program, called "My Night." Our research shows that this enables you to make healthy choices on your own.

Getting the Support You Need

Many couples join my weight management program together. Committing to a healthful lifestyle with a partner provides invaluable support. Keeping our own weight at a health-promoting level is crucial, of course—but so is helping our loved ones manage their own weight.

Of course, there can be frustration at times, as men typically lose weight faster than women. One of the primary reasons has to do with body composition. Women will always have a higher percentage of body fat, which is needed during the childbearing years to ensure proper energy conservation for pregnancy and breastfeeding. Men typically have more lean muscle tissue, which burns more calories, even at rest.

This muscle-to-fat ratio is very important, as you know. A young, athletic man needs a good amount of quality lean protein and can tolerate more carbohydrates due to his larger muscle mass and activity level. This shifts slightly as he gets older and is less active. Women, particularly after menopause, need adequate protein but also must confront a more drastically reduced tolerance to carbohydrates.

As a result, I've found it useful when working with couples to make just a few simple changes. It's important that both parties agree to work together and that health decisions are mutually agreed on. It's also important that no one turns into the food police!

Many couples often go out to eat, sharing food and drinks, as this is a highly pleasurable thing to do. As you will likely be eating out a lot less when you are in the early stages of the **MD Factor** Action Plan, try to find a non-food-related interest to share, such as a hobby or an activity (maybe bike riding or hiking). Preparing healthful food at home is also a great way to experiment and explore your talents as a cook as well as spend time together.

It's also very helpful to arrange your schedules so both partners can exercise without missing obligations or slacking on responsibilities. Families, especially those with children, typically have to work hard at time management and shared chores to be able to slot in the time to exercise while still caring for everyone else's needs.

For example, my husband and I make arrangements so I can go to the gym in the morning and he can go in the afternoon. We divide our family responsibilities—which isn't always easy when you have four children—and I try to make my husband's health time just as important as my own. Even better, if you can exercise together, celebrate what your bodies can do and get stronger as a couple.

Keep in mind that it's very easy to sabotage your own or your partner's efforts by skipping workouts or overindulging in food and drink. Do your best to support each other, because eating well and exercising regularly are the best ways to maintain your health and vitality.

> Eating well and exercising regularly are the best ways to maintain your health and vitality.

Update: Jennifer, Steve & Michelle

Now let's take a look at the three patients you read about at the beginning of this book.

Jennifer, Triumphant

It is amazing! I am at 135 pounds and thinner now than I was when I was in high school. My friends and relatives who haven't seen me in a while can't believe I look this good after having a child.

It took fourteen months to lose ninety-five pounds. I felt great during the entire process, and my energy level is amazing. I've maintained my weight loss for more than six months and have been able to come off the metformin. I'm planning to conceive this year and I know I am not going

to gain too much weight. My meal plan will be modified for my pregnancy, of course, but I will eat the same healthful foods that have become my new way of life. I will be monitored for gestational diabetes, since I have had it before, but I know I can control it.

My entire family is feeling better and my husband, Rob, lost forty pounds just because we eat better in general. We are great role models for good nutrition for our son and his friends, too.

When I was almost a hundred pounds heavier, I thought my only option was weight loss surgery. I am so happy I went to see Dr. Cederquist and her team, because I understand my metabolism now and how I need to take care of myself to stay healthy and not become diabetic like my mother. I should also be able to get pregnant now without worrying about my body having trouble absorbing vitamins, which happens after weight-loss surgeries and is a real problem during pregnancy.

Seeing Dr. Cederquist and figuring out my metabolism was one of the best decisions I have ever made.

Steve, Triumphant

I learned so much about my body and metabolism by coming to see Dr. Cederquist. I never realized how important my diet was to my health and my weight. I've always believed that if I just worked out, I could eat whatever I wanted and still keep my weight down, but clearly that was not the case with me with getting older.

I don't feel like I'm stuck on any type of diet. This is my new lifestyle. I get enough protein at all meals and snacks, and I keep an eye on my carb intake. It's easy. I still eat out at lunch, but now I just eat the right things. I am now a tried-and-true breakfast eater. Eating my snacks really helps, too. I don't get overly hungry at mealtimes if I am consistent with eating my snacks.

The most important thing is that my cholesterol profile is so much better. My good cholesterol went up. My triglycerides went into the normal range. My blood pressure is also perfect again. I didn't have to start any medications to do it, either. I lost thirty pounds and am back to a great weight for me at 190 pounds; on some of the height/weight tables the 190 may still seem high, but I am very muscular. Dr. Cederquist has confirmed that my body fat is low and where it should be, and she says the proof is in my awesome blood work. My health is back in my control and I am so grateful.

Michelle, Triumphant

I have my metabolism, my body, and my life back!

I was at wits' end when I came to see Dr. Cederquist last year. I was doing everything possible to lose weight and instead was gaining. I was working so hard and had nothing to show for it. I was getting depressed and felt my body was letting me down. I thought this is just what I have to look forward to with getting older and being postmenopausal.

When Dr. Cederquist tested my blood, she found that my cholesterol was up and so was my test of three-month blood sugar control—the HA1C. My blood pressure was also a little high at 140/90. Dr. Cederquist recommended that I not take cholesterol-lowering pills or blood pressure medication. Instead, I followed the **MD Factor** Action Plan.

She also found I was low in vitamin B12, magnesium, and vitamin D. I changed my diet to what she recommended and took my supplements. At the end of four months I was back to my perfect weight of 118. I have kept the weight off for almost a year now.

I am so thrilled. I look like myself again and have my energy back. I am no longer craving sugars. My hot flashes decreased as well and now they are very infrequent. Dr. Cederquist was very excited to see that my cholesterol level is absolutely perfect and so is my blood pressure. I am on no medications and doing well. I still work and still travel for work. Eating the right way for my metabolism is very doable. It's just not doable if you don't have the right information. And now I do!

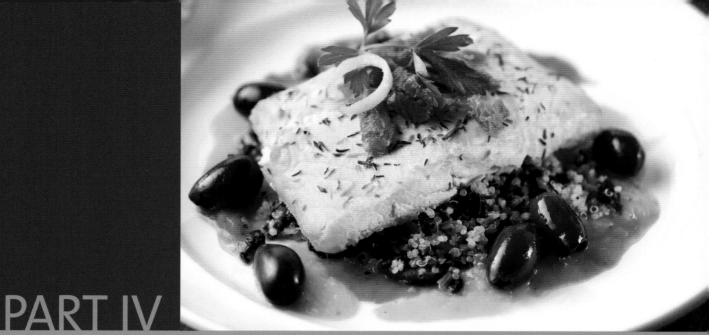

Salmon with red and yellow pepper coulis sauce

PART IV

RECIPES

Turkey Burgers and Slaw

Serves 6 | 30 grams protein | 17 grams of net carbohydrates per serving

Burger

INGREDIENTS

2 pounds lean ground turkey

1 cup oats

3 garlic cloves, minced

2 tablespoons Worcestershire sauce

1 ½ teaspoons dried oregano

1 teaspoon dried basil

dash of salt

½ teaspoon black pepper

INSTRUCTIONS

1. Preheat grill or large frying pan. Mix all ingredients together and form six ¼-inch-thick patties.
2. Cook about 6 minutes on each side.

Slaw

INGREDIENTS

½ small red cabbage and ½ small green cabbage, thinly sliced

8 radishes, thinly sliced

1 carrot, grated

1 stalk celery, chopped

dash of garlic powder

2 tablespoons of olive oil

2 teaspoons of vinegar

1 teaspoon lemon juice

INSTRUCTIONS

1. Mix all ingredients together in a bowl and allow to chill in the refrigerator.
2. Stir before serving.

Macadamia and Oat-Crusted Halibut with Sautéed Spinach

Serves 4 | 33 grams protein | 11 grams of net carbohydrates per serving

Halibut

INGREDIENTS

1 cup old-fashioned oats
½ cup macadamia nuts, chopped
1 tablespoon fresh thyme, chopped
1 teaspoon garlic, minced
dash of salt
3 tablespoons water
1 egg white
4 halibut fillets, or other white fish (4 ounces each fillet)
spritz of olive oil

INSTRUCTIONS

1. Preheat oven to 400 degrees F. Combine oats, macadamia nuts, thyme, garlic, and salt in a large dish. In another medium-size dish, beat water and egg white until frothy. Dip the halibut fillets into the egg mixture and coat the fillet. Then dip into the oat mixture and coat on both sides.

2. Spritz a casserole dish with olive oil and place the halibut fillets in the dish. Bake for 10–12 minutes or until the fish flakes easily with a fork.

Sautéed Spinach

INGREDIENTS

1 tablespoon olive oil
¼ cup onions, chopped
1 garlic clove, minced
4 cups of fresh spinach leaves
dash of salt
¼ teaspoon of white pepper

INSTRUCTIONS

1. In a large skillet, heat the olive oil on medium heat. Add in the onions and garlic until onions are translucent.

2. Add the spinach and sauté until leaves become wilted.

3. Sprinkle with salt and white pepper. Stir before serving.

Lemon Chicken Picatta with Squash Ribbons

Serves 4 | 32 grams protein | 20 grams of net carbohydrates per serving

Chicken

INGREDIENTS

4 boneless, skinless chicken breast fillets (about 4–5 ounces each)

2 tablespoons olive oil

1 large sweet onion, chopped

2 garlic cloves, minced

¼ cup all-purpose flour

dash of salt

1 cup low-sodium chicken broth

juice of 2 lemons

1 tablespoon capers

2 tablespoons fresh parsley, finely chopped

INSTRUCTIONS

1. Pat each chicken breast dry.

2. Place a piece of plastic wrap across a cutting board. Then, lay the chicken breast on top of the plastic wrap and place another piece of plastic wrap over the chicken. Using a mallet, flatten the chicken breast until it is about 1/4" thick. Repeat with remaining 3 breasts.

3. Heat a large sauté pan over medium-high heat and add the olive oil.

4. Add the onion and garlic to the sauté pan and cook until onions are translucent, about 2 minutes. Remove from pan and set aside.

5. In a shallow, elongated dish, combine the flour and a dash of salt.

6. Coat both sides of the chicken breast with the flour mix and add them one at a time to the hot pan. Cook 2–3 minutes per side or until they are golden brown.

7. Remove chicken breasts from pan and set aside on a plate.

8. To make the sauce, add the chicken broth, lemon juice, capers, and previously sautéed onion and garlic to the pan and heat.

9. Return the chicken to the pan, bring the liquid to a boil, lower the heat, and simmer for about 3 minutes or until the mixture has reduced. Add the chopped parsley at the end and serve.

Squash Ribbons

INGREDIENTS

2 medium zucchini

2 medium yellow squash

½ tablespoon olive oil

½ teaspoon garlic, minced

dash of red pepper flakes

½ teaspoon salt

⅛ teaspoon black pepper

sprinkle of Parmesan cheese, reduced fat

INSTRUCTIONS

1. Cut zucchini and squash thinly using a vegetable peeler down the length of the squash.

2. In a large sauté pan on medium heat, add the olive oil, garlic, and red pepper flakes.

3. Add the zucchini, squash, salt and pepper and cook for 3–4 minutes until tender. Sprinkle with reduced-fat Parmesan cheese and serve.

Pork Chops with Onion-Mushroom Gravy and Cauliflower Mash

| Serves 4 | 34 grams protein | 13 grams of net carbohydrates per serving |

Pork Chops

INGREDIENTS

1 pound of button mushrooms, thinly sliced

2 medium shallots, thinly sliced

2 garlic cloves, thinly sliced

spritz of olive oil

4 boneless center cut pork chops, fat trimmed (5 ounces each)

1 ½ cups low-sodium beef stock or vegetable broth

3 sprigs of fresh thyme

1 tablespoon olive oil

black pepper, to taste

INSTRUCTIONS

1. Preheat large sauté pan over medium-high heat.
2. Clean and slice mushrooms.
3. Add mushrooms to the dry pan and cook for about 4 minutes until caramelized.
4. Slice shallots and garlic and set aside.
5. Remove mushrooms from pan and set aside.
6. Spritz pan with olive oil and add shallots and garlic to the pan. Cook for 2–3 minutes or until caramelized. Remove from pan and set aside with the mushrooms.
7. Add the pork chops to the pan and brown both sides, about 5 minutes per side. Remove the pork and set aside.
8. Increase the heat of the pan to high and add stock to pan and stir.
9. Reduce heat to medium. Add the thyme and allow the stock to reduce by half.
10. Return pork chops to the pan and reduce heat to low. Cover and cook the pork for 5 minutes or until the pork is fully cooked through.
11. Remove pork chops and set aside. Discard the thyme stems. Add olive oil to the pan and stir until well combined. Then add mushrooms, shallots, and garlic. Stir together in the pan to make the gravy. Add black pepper to taste.
12. Pour the gravy over the pork chops and serve.

Cauliflower Mash

INGREDIENTS

1 head of cauliflower, cut into large florets

4 garlic cloves

1 (14-ounce) can of reduced-sodium chicken broth

2 ounces of cream cheese, reduced fat

salt and black pepper, to taste

chives, to taste

INSTRUCTIONS

1. Combine cauliflower, garlic, and broth in a large saucepan and bring to a boil.
2. Reduce heat to low and simmer for 15 minutes.
3. Remove cauliflower from the pan and drain.
4. Place the cauliflower and garlic in a food processor and blend until smooth.
5. If needed, add 1 tablespoon of the chicken broth until desired consistency.
6. Add in the cream cheese and season with salt and black pepper to taste.
7. Fold in chives and serve.

Stuffed Chicken with Green Bean and Tomato Salad

| Serves 4 | 32 grams protein | 8 grams of net carbohydrates per serving |

Chicken

INGREDIENTS

2 ounces of Canadian bacon, diced

4 light Laughing Cow cheese wedges, garlic and herb flavored

4 boneless, skinless chicken breasts (about 4–5 ounces each)

black pepper, to taste

INSTRUCTIONS

1. Preheat oven to 400 degrees F.
2. Combine the diced Canadian bacon and light Laughing Cow cheese wedges in a bowl and mix together.
3. Cut a slit in each chicken breast to form a pocket and stuff about 2 tablespoons of the cheese mixture into each breast. Close the opening with a toothpick, if needed. Sprinkle with black pepper.
4. Bake for 30–35 minutes or until the chicken is cooked through.

Green Bean and Tomato Salad

INGREDIENTS

2 cups fresh green beans, trimmed

1 cup cherry tomatoes, cut in half

1 red bell pepper, thinly sliced

¼ cup red onion, sliced

2 garlic cloves, minced

1 tablespoon olive oil

1 tablespoon balsamic vinegar

salt and black pepper, to taste

INSTRUCTIONS

1. Using a small saucepan, boil green beans for 5 minutes or until al dente.
2. Drain water, place green beans in a medium-size bowl and set aside.
3. Once the green beans are cooled to room temperature, add the cherry tomatoes, red bell pepper, onion, garlic, olive oil, balsamic vinegar, and salt and black pepper. Mix together until all ingredients are evenly combined.
4. Let marinate in refrigerator for 30 minutes to 1 hour and serve cold.

Chicken Cacciatore with Italian Green Beans

Serves 4 | 29 grams protein | 18 grams of net carbohydrates per serving

Chicken Cacciatore

INGREDIENTS

spritz of olive oil

1 pound boneless, skinless chicken breast

1 yellow onion, diced

1 green bell pepper, cut into 1-inch pieces

1 red bell pepper, cut into 1-inch pieces

2 garlic cloves, minced

1 (28-ounce) can, diced tomatoes, no salt added

3 tablespoons capers, drained and rinsed

1 teaspoon dried oregano

1 teaspoon dried basil

salt and black pepper, to taste

INSTRUCTIONS

1. Heat a large skillet to medium-high heat and spritz with olive oil.

2. Add the chicken to the skillet and cook until browned and cooked through.

3. Once cooked through, remove the chicken from the skillet and place on a plate. Add the onions, bell peppers, and garlic to the skillet and cook over medium heat until onions are translucent.

4. Add the tomatoes, capers, oregano, basil, and salt and black pepper to taste and mix.

5. Return the chicken to the skillet and increase the heat to high to bring contents to a boil.

6. Reduce heat to low. Cover and simmer for 30 minutes.

Italian Green Beans

INGREDIENTS

1 teaspoon olive oil

1 garlic clove, minced

1 pound Italian flat beans, frozen

1 tablespoon Italian seasoning

salt and black pepper, to taste

INSTRUCTIONS

1. Heat oil over medium heat in a medium sauté pan. Add the garlic and sauté for 2 minutes.

2. Add the flat beats and continue to cook for about 5 minutes.

3. Add the Italian seasoning and salt and black pepper to taste and continue cooking until beans are al dente.

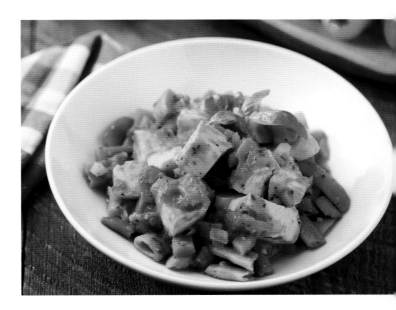

Lemon and Rosemary Chicken with Turkey Bacon Brussels Sprouts

Serves 4 | 34 grams protein | 7 grams of net carbohydrates per serving

Chicken

INGREDIENTS

4 garlic cloves, minced

4 tablespoons fresh rosemary, chopped

4 tablespoons lemon juice

2 teaspoons lemon zest

salt and black pepper, to taste

4 boneless, skinless chicken breasts
   (about 4–5 ounces each)

INSTRUCTIONS

1. Preheat the oven to 375 degrees F.
2. Using a food processor, pulse the garlic, rosemary, lemon juice, lemon zest, salt and pepper until blended.
3. Coat each chicken breast with the mixture and place them in a baking dish.
4. Bake for 25–30 minutes or until juices run clear.

Brussels Sprouts

INGREDIENTS

2 tablespoons olive oil

1 pound of Brussels sprouts, trimmed and cut in half

salt and black pepper, to taste

4 slices of turkey bacon

1 cup of chicken broth, low sodium

zest of 1 lemon

INSTRUCTIONS

1. Heat a large sauté pan over medium heat. Add the olive oil and the Brussels sprouts and sauté until lightly browned. Add salt and black pepper to taste.
2. In the meantime, cook the 4 slices of turkey bacon.
3. Add the chicken broth to the Brussels sprouts, turn the heat to low, and cook uncovered for about 15 minutes or until Brussels sprouts are tender.
4. Remove from the pan and place in a serving dish. Crumble the turkey bacon on top with the lemon zest and serve.

Spaghetti Squash and Chicken and Vegetable Stuffing

Serves 2 | 32 grams protein | 18 grams of net carbohydrates per serving

INGREDIENTS

1 spaghetti squash, cut in half lengthwise, seeds removed

1 teaspoon olive oil

2 boneless, skinless chicken breasts (about 4–5 ounces each)

2 small yellow onions, chopped

3 garlic cloves, minced

4 plum tomatoes, diced

1 green bell pepper, diced

1 red bell pepper, diced

1 cup fresh mushrooms, sliced

¼ cup tomato puree

2 tablespoons fresh basil, chopped

1 tablespoon oregano

1 tablespoon parsley, fresh

3 tablespoons mozzarella cheese, reduced fat, shredded

3 tablespoons Parmesan cheese, reduced fat, grated

INSTRUCTIONS

1. Preheat the oven to 375 degrees F. Cut the spaghetti squash in half lengthwise and place cut side down on a baking sheet. Bake for 40–45 minutes or until the squash can be easily pierced with a fork.

2. Set aside the squash and allow it to cool.

3. Heat a large saucepan over medium heat and add the olive oil.

4. Cut the chicken into small chunks and add to the saucepan. Cook until browned and cooked through. Remove from pan and set aside.

5. Add the onions to the saucepan and sauté until translucent, then add the garlic and sauté one minute.

6. Add the tomatoes, bell peppers, mushrooms, tomato puree, basil, oregano, and parsley. Simmer for 20 minutes.

7. Once the squash is cool enough to handle, use a fork to separate the squash into strands. Keep the hollowed squash halves.

8. Place the spaghetti strands in a large bowl and add the sautéed vegetable mixture and chicken. Mix all ingredients together.

9. Use the hollowed squash halves and stuff each half with the mixture and place on a baking sheet.

10. Top each stuffed squash with the mozzarella and Parmesan.

11. Bake in the oven until the cheese is melted and slightly brown, about 15 minutes.

Old-Fashioned Beef Stew

Serves 4 | 31 grams protein
13 grams of net carbohydrates per serving

INGREDIENTS

1 pound boneless top sirloin

1 large sweet onion, diced

2 cups mushrooms, sliced

4 garlic cloves, chopped

drizzle of olive oil

2 teaspoons tomato paste

2 cups reduced-sodium beef broth

4 cups sliced carrots

1 cup green beans, cut into 1-inch pieces

1 teaspoon cornstarch

1 teaspoon cold water

½ cup fresh parsley

INSTRUCTIONS

1. Dice sirloin into small cubes and cook in a large sauté pan until cooked through.

2. In a large soup pot add the onions, mushrooms, garlic, and a drizzle of olive oil and sauté for about 5 minutes.

3. Add the cooked beef to the onion and mushroom mixture and stir in the tomato paste and beef broth.

4. Add enough water to just cover the contents. Bring to a boil.

5. Add the carrots and green beans. Cover the pot partially and simmer for 30 minutes.

6. In a separate bowl, mix the cornstarch and cold water together and then stir into the stew.

7. Increase heat of the stew and boil uncovered for 1 minute or until stew thickens.

8. Ladle into soup bowls and garnish with fresh parsley.

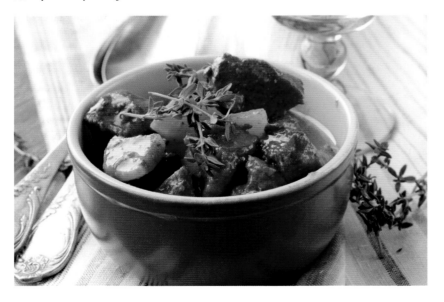

Grilled Mediterranean Kabobs

Serves 2 | 30 grams protein
12 grams of net carbohydrates per 2 skewer serving

INGREDIENTS

2 (12-ounce) cans artichoke hearts, packed in water, cut in half

2 red, orange, or yellow bell peppers, cut into 1-inch pieces

8 green olives

1 package fully cooked chicken sausage, cut into 1-inch pieces

4 wooden skewers

½ cup light Italian dressing

INSTRUCTIONS

1. Slide the vegetables, green olives, and chicken sausage pieces onto water-soaked wooden skewers, dividing the ingredients equally among each skewer.

2. Place kabobs in a baking dish and drizzle with Italian dressing to marinate.

3. Place the kabobs on the grill until heated through, rotating every couple of minutes.

NOTES

- Serve over a bed of fresh salad greens if enjoying on the Reclaim Phase.

- You may serve with ½ cup cooked quinoa, ½ cup cooked brown rice, ½ cup of cooked beans, or ¼ cup hummus as a healthy complex carb for both transformation and stabilization phases.

Breakfast Frittata

Serves 6 | 16 grams of protein
4 grams of net carbohydrate per serving

INGREDIENTS

1 (10-ounce) package chopped, frozen spinach

spritz of olive oil

1 teaspoon olive oil

3 teaspoons raw onion, minced

4 fully cooked chicken sausage links, diced into small pieces

2 whole eggs

1 cup egg whites

1 cup cheese, reduced fat

INSTRUCTIONS

1. Preheat the oven to 350 degrees F. Thaw spinach and drain the excess water.

2. Spritz a pie pan with olive oil.

3. In a small skillet over medium heat, heat the teaspoon of olive oil, then add in the onion, sauté until translucent, and set aside.

4. In a mixing bowl, beat the eggs and egg whites.

5. To the eggs, add the onion, sausage, spinach, and cheese.

6. Pour mixture into pie pan and bake for 20–30 minutes until the eggs set.

Eggplant Rollatini

Serves 4 | 24 grams protein
25 grams net carbohydrates per serving

INGREDIENTS

spritz of olive oil

1 large eggplant, cut lengthwise into 8 slices

1 (10-ounce) package of chopped, frozen spinach, thawed and squeezed to remove excess water

1 ½ cups reduced-fat ricotta cheese

½ cup fresh basil, chopped

2 eggs, whisked or ¼ cup egg substitute

2 cloves garlic, chopped

¼ teaspoon black pepper

⅛ teaspoon salt

2 cups marinara sauce

1 cup part-skim mozzarella cheese, shredded

INSTRUCTIONS

1. Preheat oven to 350 degrees F. Spritz 2 baking sheets and a 9-by-13-inch baking dish with olive oil.

2. Place the sliced eggplant onto the baking sheets and bake 10 minutes, and then flip the slices and bake another 10 minutes.

3. While the eggplant bakes, mix spinach, ricotta cheese, basil, egg, garlic, pepper, and salt in a large bowl.

4. Remove the eggplant from the oven and distribute spinach-ricotta mixture among the bottoms of the eggplant slices and roll up each slice around the mixture. Place the rolled eggplant pieces in the baking dish, seam-side down.

5. Liberally cover the rolls in the baking dish with marinara sauce. Cover pan with aluminum foil and bake for 20 minutes.

6. Remove foil and sprinkle rolls with mozzarella cheese. Bake uncovered, until cheese has melted and is bubbling, about 10–15 minutes.

Curry Chicken Salad

Serves 4 | 27 grams protein
8 grams net carbohydrates per serving

INGREDIENTS

1 pound of boneless, skinless chicken breast

¼ cup reduced-fat plain Greek yogurt

¼ cup reduced-fat sour cream

1 teaspoon of curry powder, or to taste

½ cup apple, diced

½ cup mango, diced

½ cup celery, diced

1 tablespoon fresh cilantro, chopped

1 teaspoon scallion, chopped

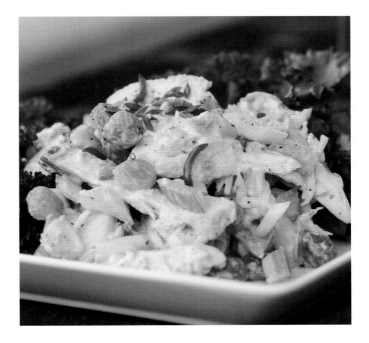

INSTRUCTIONS

1. Place chicken breast in a medium sauce pan and add just enough water to cover the chicken. Bring the water to a boil and let boil for about 15 minutes until chicken is cooked through.

2. Remove from heat, drain the water, and allow chicken to cool.

3. In a large bowl, whisk together Greek yogurt, sour cream, and curry powder. Set aside.

4. Add the diced apple, mango, celery, cilantro, and scallion to the yogurt mixture.

5. Once chicken has cooled, dice into small pieces and add to the yogurt and fruit mixture. Toss all ingredients until thoroughly combined. Cover bowl and chill in refrigerator until ready to serve.

6. Enjoy on a bed of greens.

Sides

These delicious sides and the sauces that follow can be combined with any lean protein choice for delicious and endless combinations.

Swiss Chard and Tomato Sauté

Serves 4–6	3 grams of protein
5 grams of net carbohydrate per 1 cup serving	

INGREDIENTS

1 pound red Swiss chard
1 tablespoon olive oil
1 garlic clove, minced
dash of red pepper flakes
2 small tomatoes, diced
dash of salt

INSTRUCTIONS

1. Separate the stems of the Swiss chard from the leaves.
2. Cut the stems and the leaves into ½-inch slices.
3. Heat 1 tablespoon of olive oil in a large skillet. Add garlic and red pepper flakes and stir occasionally for 1–2 minutes.
4. Add the stems and cook until tender, about 6–7 minutes.
5. Add the Swiss chard leaves and cook until slightly wilted, about 1–2 minutes.
6. Add the tomatoes and dash of salt. Cook until heated through and then serve.

Edamame and Artichoke Salad

Serves about 9 | 7 grams of protein
6 grams of net carbohydrate per ½ cup serving

INGREDIENTS

1 (16-ounce) package frozen edamame, shelled

1 tablespoon olive oil

4 shallots, thinly sliced

1 (14-ounce) can of artichoke hearts, packed in water

¼ cup sun-dried tomatoes

¼ cup fresh-squeezed lemon juice

INSTRUCTIONS

1. Heat the shelled edamame in the microwave for about 2 minutes, until heated through.
2. Heat the olive oil in a large skillet over medium heat and add the shallots. Cook until slightly brown and soft.
3. Chop the artichoke hearts in half and place in a medium-size bowl. Add the cooked edamame, shallots, sun-dried tomatoes, and lemon juice. Stir to evenly combine all ingredients and serve.

Dill Cucumber Salad

Serves approx 3 | 2 grams of protein
5 grams of net carbohydrate per 1 cup serving

INGREDIENTS

2 large cucumbers, peeled and thinly sliced

2 scallions, thinly sliced

1 tablespoon lemon juice

¼ cup low-fat plain yogurt

¼ teaspoon garlic powder

¼ teaspoon salt

black pepper, to taste

INSTRUCTIONS

1. Combine all ingredients in a large bowl and mix.
2. Cover with plastic wrap and refrigerate until ready to serve.

Cauliflower Rice

Serves 6 | 3 grams of protein
4 grams of net carbohydrate per 1 cup serving

INGREDIENTS

3 tablespoons olive oil

1 medium yellow onion, diced

1 cup celery, finely diced

1 head of cauliflower, trimmed and coarsely chopped

¼ teaspoon salt

INSTRUCTIONS

1. In a large skillet, heat olive oil over medium heat.
2. Sauté onion over medium heat until translucent.
3. Add celery and sauté for 5 minutes.
4. Meanwhile, pulse the cauliflower in a food processor until it develops the texture of rice.
5. Add cauliflower to the skillet, cover, and cook 5–10 minutes, until soft. Add salt or other seasonings to taste.

Zucchini Pasta

Serves 4 | 3 grams of protein
4 grams of net carbohydrate per 1 cup serving

INGREDIENTS

2 pounds zucchini

2 tablespoons olive oil

salt and black pepper, to taste

¾ cup tomato sauce (optional)

¼ cup reduced-fat Parmesan cheese, grated (optional)

INSTRUCTIONS

1. Using a vegetable peeler, cut zucchini into lengthwise ribbons. Peel off several from one side, then turn the zucchini and peel off more. Continue to turn and peel away ribbons until you get to the seeds at the core of the zucchini. Discard the core. You may also do this on a mandolin, adjusted to a very thin slice.
2. Cook zucchini strips in two batches. Heat 1 tablespoon of the oil in a large skillet over medium-high heat. When hot, add the zucchini ribbons and a dash of salt. Cook by tossing the zucchini for 2–3 minutes, until softened and beginning to turn translucent. Add additional salt and black pepper to taste.
3. Transfer to a serving dish and repeat with remaining olive oil and zucchini.
4. Serve, topping with tomato sauce and Parmesan, if desired.
5. This dish is best served right away. However, enjoy leftovers with lemon juice and a drop of olive oil.

Tomato Tabbouleh

Serves 6　|　2 grams of protein
5 grams of net carbohydrate per ¼ cup serving

INGREDIENTS

1 cup baby vine tomatoes, deseeded, diced, and drained

1 cup flat leaf parsley, rough chopped

¼ cup raw sesame seeds

4 tablespoons olive oil

juice from 2 lemons

4 teaspoons local honey

INSTRUCTIONS

1. Place tomatoes in a bowl and stir in the parsley and sesame seeds. Whisk together the remaining ingredients and drizzle onto the tomato mixture and toss together.

Roasted Cauliflower with Pesto

Serves 4　|　2 grams of protein
2 grams of net carbohydrate per 1 cup serving

INGREDIENTS

1 head of cauliflower, cut into bite-size florets

3 tablespoons olive oil

salt and black pepper, to taste

3 tablespoons pesto, homemade or store bought

INSTRUCTIONS

1. Preheat oven to 425 degrees F.
2. Toss the cauliflower with olive oil. Spread on a parchment lined baking sheet, sprinkle with salt and black pepper.
3. Roast until golden brown and tender.
4. Transfer to a serving bowl and add pesto. Toss and serve.

French Lentil Salad

Serves 8 | 6 grams of protein
10 grams of net carbohydrate per 1/2 cup serving

INGREDIENTS

1 tablespoon olive oil

1 cup white onion, diced

½ cup carrot, diced

½ cup celery, diced

2 cloves garlic, minced

2 tablespoons white cooking wine

1 (18-ounce) package cooked French lentils

¼ cup low-sodium chicken stock

salt and black pepper, to taste

INSTRUCTIONS

1. In a medium sauté pan, heat the olive oil on medium heat. Add the onions, carrots, and celery and sauté until soft, about 5–7 minutes. Add the garlic and cook another 2 minutes.

2. Deglaze the pan with white wine and allow to boil for 1–2 minutes.

3. Add French lentils until warm.

4. Add the chicken stock to moisten the lentils, but not drench. Add salt and black pepper to taste.

White Beans with Pesto

Serves 11 | 6 grams of protein
14 grams of net carbohydrate per 1/2 cup serving

INGREDIENTS

1 tablespoon olive oil

1 white onion, diced

2 garlic cloves, minced

2 tablespoons white cooking wine

2 (14.5-ounce) cans cannellini beans, drained and rinsed

½ cup pesto, homemade or store bought

2 tablespoons sun-dried tomatoes, chopped

salt, to taste

INSTRUCTIONS

1. In a medium sauté pan over medium heat, add the olive oil and sauté onions until translucent.

2. Add the garlic and cook another 2 minutes.

3. Deglaze the pan with white wine and allow to boil for 1–2 minutes.

4. Add cannellini beans, pesto, and sun-dried tomatoes and heat until warm throughout.

5. Add salt to taste and serve.

Edamame Caviar

Serves 8 | 5 grams of protein
6 grams of net carbohydrate per ½ cup serving

INGREDIENTS

2 cups frozen shelled edamame, thawed
½ cup carrot, finely diced
½ cup zucchini, finely diced
1 red bell pepper, finely diced
½ cup yellow corn kernels
½ cup red onion, finely diced
1 garlic clove, minced
¼ cup fresh parsley, chopped
2 tablespoons fresh basil, chopped

Dressing

⅓ cup fresh lemon juice
2 tablespoons Dijon mustard
2 tablespoons olive oil
¾ teaspoon sea salt
¾ teaspoon black pepper

INSTRUCTIONS

1. Prepare edamame according to package directions. Drain and rinse with cold water. Set aside to drain thoroughly.

2. Combine all ingredients except the dressing. Mix gently.

3. In a separate bowl, whisk together dressing ingredients. Slowly add dressing to the vegetable mix until covered to desired amount. Refrigerate until ready to serve.

Ratatouille

Serves 8 | 1 gram of protein
3 grams of net carbohydrate per ½ cup serving

INGREDIENTS

1 teaspoon olive oil
1 green bell pepper, diced
2 cups eggplant, diced
1 zucchini, diced
1 (14.5-ounce) can diced tomato, fire roasted
1 teaspoon fresh thyme, chopped
salt and black pepper, to taste

INSTRUCTIONS

1. In a sauté pan, heat 1 teaspoon of olive oil over medium heat. When oil is heated, add the bell pepper, eggplant, and zucchini and sauté for about 10 minutes, until vegetables become soft.

2. Add the diced tomatoes and thyme, turn the heat to medium-low, cover, and let simmer for another 10 minutes. Add salt and black pepper to taste.

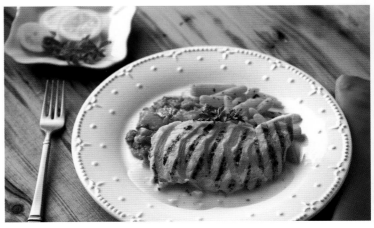

Grilled chicken breast with garlic velouté ratatouille and carrots

Sauces, Toppings, Salad Dressings

These flavorful combinations can be combined with any lean protein choice.

Pineapple Salsa

Serves 8 | 1 gram of protein
4 grams of net carbohydrate per $1/2$ cup serving

INGREDIENTS

2 ½ cups tomatoes, diced

½ cup red onion, diced

½ cup pineapple, diced

1 red chili, deseeded and diced (optional)

½ garlic clove, finely chopped

2 tablespoons olive oil

juice from one lime

INSTRUCTIONS

1. Place all ingredients in a bowl and toss until thoroughly combined.

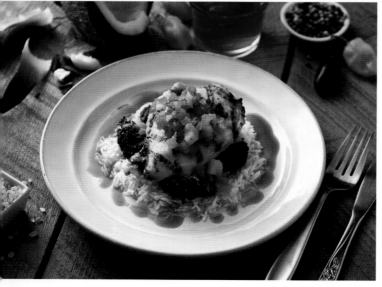

Grilled chicken with pineapple salsa topping

Mango Salsa

Serves 5 | 1 gram of protein
6 grams of net carbohydrate per ¼ cup serving

INGREDIENTS

1 ripe mango, diced

2 tablespoons fresh cilantro, chopped

1 jalapeno, diced (optional)

¼ cup red bell pepper, diced

¼ teaspoon ground cumin

1 tablespoon lime juice

salt, to taste

INSTRUCTIONS

1. Place all of the ingredients together in a mixing bowl and gently toss until combined. Refrigerate until ready to serve.

Tahini Salad Dressing

Serves 6 | 2 grams of protein
3 grams of net carbohydrate per 2 tablespoon serving

INGREDIENTS

¼ cup tahini

2 tablespoons low-sodium soy sauce

1 tablespoon red wine vinegar

1 tablespoon lemon juice

1 teaspoon fresh ginger, minced

1 garlic clove, minced

¼ cup Italian dressing, reduced fat

INSTRUCTIONS

1. Blend all ingredients up to Italian dressing in a blender or food processor until smooth. Slowly add the Italian dressing until you reach a desired consistency and flavor.

Garlic Velouté

| Serves 6 | 1 gram of protein |
4 grams of net carbohydrate per ¼ cup serving

INGREDIENTS

2 heads of garlic

olive oil, a few drops to oil pan

1 teaspoon flour

1 ½ cups low-sodium chicken stock

salt and black pepper, to taste

INSTRUCTIONS

1. Cut the base of the head of garlic, wrap it in aluminum foil and bake at 400 degrees F for 30–35 minutes, until tender. Let cool slightly then remove the foil and extract the roasted garlic paste.

2. Heat a sauté pan with a few drops of olive oil and add the garlic paste. Stir as you sprinkle in the flour. Stir again and let cook for a few second. Moisten with the chicken stock and cook until it reaches the desired texture. Season to taste with salt and pepper.

Marsala Sauce

| Serves 9 | 1 gram of protein |
2 grams of net carbohydrate per ¼ cup serving

INGREDIENTS

1 tablespoon olive oil

¼ cup white onion, diced

1 clove garlic, chopped

½ pound mushrooms, washed and sliced

1 tablespoon flour

¼ cup Marsala wine

¾ cup low-sodium beef stock

salt and black pepper, to taste

INSTRUCTIONS

1. Add olive oil to a medium sauce pan and heat over medium heat. When heated, add onions and garlic and cook until onions become translucent.

2. Add the mushrooms and sauté until tender.

3. Add flour and cook for about 1 minute, and then deglaze the pan with Marsala wine.

4. Add the beef stock and cook until thickened. Season with salt and pepper to taste.

Pepper Coulis

Serves 6 | 1 gram of protein
2 grams of net carbohydrate per ¼ cup serving

INGREDIENTS

2 large red bell peppers

3 tablespoons olive oil

1 medium shallot, thinly sliced

1 tablespoon red wine vinegar

salt and white pepper, to taste

INSTRUCTIONS

1. Roast the red bell peppers under the broiler, turning occasionally until the peppers are blackened all over.

2. Transfer the peppers to a bowl and let cool completely. Once cooled, peel the peppers and discard the skins, seeds, and cores, and then coarsely chop.

3. In a food processor, combine the peppers with the olive oil, shallot, and vinegar and puree until smooth. Season the coulis with salt and white pepper as desired.

Pomodoro Sauce

Serves 5 | 1 gram of protein
2 grams of net carbohydrate per ¼ cup serving

INGREDIENTS

2 garlic cloves, minced

2 tablespoons yellow onion, diced

2 tablespoons olive oil

2 tomatoes, chopped

3 tablespoons of fresh herbs (oregano, basil, parsley), chopped

salt and black pepper, to taste

INSTRUCTIONS

1. In a saucepan over medium heat, sauté garlic and onion in the olive oil for about 2 minutes.

2. Add the tomatoes and herbs and continue to cook for about 5 minutes until the tomatoes soften. Season with salt and black pepper.

Red Thai Curry Sauce

Serves 5 | 1 gram of protein
2 grams of net carbohydrate per ¼ cup serving

INGREDIENTS

2 tablespoons olive oil

2 tablespoons Thai red curry paste

1 cup unsweetened light coconut milk

1 lime, juiced

INSTRUCTIONS

1. Place a small sauce pan over medium heat and add olive oil. Stir the red curry paste into the pan until aromatic.

2. Slowly pour in the coconut milk and continue stirring. Add the lime juice and cook for about 5–10 minutes to thicken.

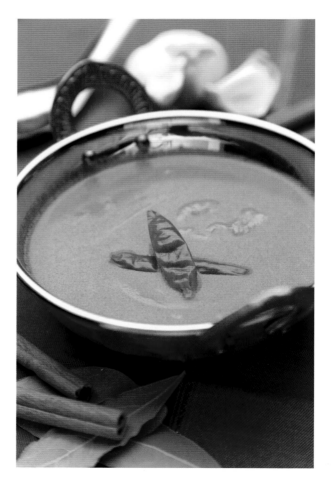

*The **MD Factor** Diet*

Baked Kale Chips

Serves 4 | 3 grams of protein
6 grams of net carbohydrate per cup serving

INGREDIENTS

1 bunch/bag of kale (about 5 cups)

spritz of olive oil

salt or seasoning to taste (chili flakes, paprika, cayenne pepper, garlic powder)

INSTRUCTIONS

1. Preheat oven to 350 degrees F.
2. Line a baking sheet with parchment paper.
3. With a knife or kitchen shears, carefully remove the leaves from the thick stems and tear into bite size pieces. Wash and thoroughly dry kale. Spritz with olive oil until leaves have a nice coating and sprinkle with desired seasonings.
4. Bake until the edges brown but are not burnt, about 10–15 minutes.

Edamole High-Protein Guacamole

Serves 4 | 17 grams of protein
9 grams of net carbohydrate per serving

INGREDIENTS

2 cups of frozen edamame, shelled and thawed

1 teaspoon salt

2 limes, juiced

dash of cayenne pepper

1 teaspoon cumin

¼ cup fresh cilantro, chopped

1 garlic clove

¼ of a sweet onion

INSTRUCTIONS

1. Combine all ingredients in a food processor and blend until smooth.
2. Serve with raw vegetables of your choice.

APPENDICES

Appendix A   Why Other Diets Don't Work

Your local bookstore has shelves laden with diet books, all claiming that their method is the best way to lose weight and keep it off. If these diets plans truly worked, however, there wouldn't be such an obesity crisis in this country—and even more diet books wouldn't be published. The fact that there's so much erroneous information out there is one of the reasons I became determined to write this book.

In this appendix, I'll explain the pros and cons of some of the most popular diets, so you will be armed with information about why the **MD Factor** Action Plan, with its far more controlled and effective way to reverse your **MD Factor**, really can help you lose weight.

Why Other Diets Don't Work Like the **MD Factor** Action Plan

Basically, the only difference from one diet to the next is the percentage of protein, carbohydrates, and fat allowed. Protein requirements are what so many others get wrong, in part due to the lasting influence of the now-retired Food Guide Pyramid.

As you read in Chapter 4, the Food Guide Pyramid was created using data from young men in the military. Their high activity level and youth meant they needed a lot of high-calorie carbohydrates to burn for energy. Unfortunately, this way of eating was not calibrated to work for people who have the **MD Factor** and whose metabolic needs are different. If you have the **MD Factor** and follow the Food Guide Pyramid's recommendations, you will be severely underestimating the amount of lean protein you need, even if you decrease calories in the hope of losing weight.

	Woman (55 years)	Man (55 years)
USDA Recommendation: Calories	1,768	2,762
USDA Recommendation: % of Calories from Protein	11.5%	12.1%
USDA Recommendation: Protein	51 grams	84 grams
MD Factor Action Plan Recommendation: Protein	100–120 grams	120–140 grams

Pretty shocking, isn't it? According to the **MD Factor** Action Plan, you should be eating more than double the amount of protein the USDA recommends. No wonder you have trouble losing weight!

Next, take a look at the **MD Factor** Action Plan compared to the Ornish Diet, the Zone Diet, and the Atkins Diet.

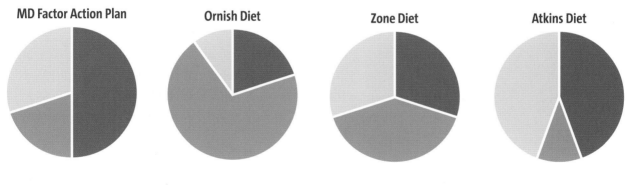

The Ornish Diet is primarily vegetarian and high in carbohydrates.

The Zone Diet is also high in carbohydrates for those with the **MD Factor**. These amounts may, however, be well tolerated for long-term weight maintenance once you've gotten down to your target weight.

On the Atkins Diet, most of your calories come from either protein or fat, and almost none from carbohydrates. Many people with the **MD Factor** find that they can lose weight on the Atkins Diet because this ratio means that muscle tissue is not broken down with weight loss. Men tend to be more successful with the Atkins Diet because they can eat so many more calories than women and still lose weight; women may lose weight initially and then plateau. What I find worrying about this diet is the high level of saturated fat allowed. With the **MD Factor** Action Plan, you eat high-quality lean protein low in saturated fat, coupled with a controlled carbohydrate intake.

Safety Concerns about High-Protein Diets

Over the years, there have been critics of high-protein diets—and many of these critics have been misinformed about how protein affects your organs and metabolism. It's time to debunk their errors!

Kidney Disease

Those suffering from kidney disease have a more difficult time clearing large particles, which includes proteins and protein by-products. As a result, if you have kidney disease, you must check with your physician before making any significant changes to your protein intake or starting any new diet.

If your kidney function is normal, increasing your protein intake will have positive effects. When you eat enough protein, your kidneys are actually able to clear waste particles more efficiently. In addition, an adequate protein intake protects your kidney function as you age.

Bone Health

High-protein diets have been criticized as being bad for your bones because they lead to a higher excretion of calcium in your urine. While this is true, the other part of the equation is that a diet adequate in protein allows greater calcium absorption from food and higher bone mineral density. In fact, there are three main contributors to strong bone density: adequate protein intake (which is the most important), physical activity, and calcium intake.

Your body likes to function in a slightly more alkaline environment. When you consume grains, they cause your body to become more acidic. This directly relates to bone health, as your bones are your body's biggest storage depot for alkaline calcium. When your body needs this calcium but is too acidic, you'll break down bone and muscle tissue to alkalinize your system. In other words, the more grains you eat, the more likely you are to break your bones!

Diets high in animal protein may also make your body more acidic, which can be a concern for bone health. The best way to make your body more alkaline is to have a high intake of vegetables. That is exactly how you eat on the **MD Factor** Action Plan—adequate lean protein with the majority of your carbs coming from vegetables.

Higher Fat Intake

In Chapter 4, you learned that your body can absorb only a specific amount of amino acids at one meal. When you eat more than you need, you won't use the excess for building and repair. Instead, it will be converted to glucose for energy—or stored as fat.

The challenge when deciding which protein to eat is to avoid foods that are also high in fat. For example, a hamburger typically contains as much fat as protein; peanut butter has almost twice as much fat as it does protein (2 tablespoons contain a whopping 190–210 calories for only 8 grams of protein, so you'd need to eat 760–800 calories of peanut butter in order to reach the necessary 30 grams of protein!). On the other hand, a serving of most fish, excluding salmon, has very little fat—in most cases, less than 2 grams in a 4-ounce serving. The fat in salmon is also healthful, as it consists of omega-3 fatty acids.

For a list of lean protein sources, see the chart "Protein Portions" in Chapter 11.

You don't need to entirely avoid protein sources with higher fat. For example, a slice of bacon adds a lot of flavor to an egg white omelet, but a whole egg omelet with lots of bacon will give you too much protein and fat. An alternative to bacon is Canadian bacon, which is a lot leaner but still adds a lot of flavor.

Cholesterol Levels

You likely already know that foods such as eggs, shrimp, and high-fat meats are high in cholesterol. But your body's production of cholesterol and the level of saturated fat in a food are much more important than a food's actual cholesterol content.

Genetics play a huge factor in the amount of cholesterol particles floating through your bloodstream, but new research shows that sugar may also be a large and surprising factor. Cholesterol levels typically go up when weight goes up, but scientists are not yet sure why sugars increase these levels, especially as they often lower your good HDL cholesterol levels at the same time. This may be partly due to the presence of fructose, which has been shown to increase new lipid creation in the liver and the secretion of LDL or "bad" cholesterol.

My patients with the **MD Factor** often have elevated total cholesterol levels combined with low "good" (HDL) cholesterol. After about six weeks on the **MD Factor** Action Plan, their cholesterol levels decrease significantly and often become normal. HDL levels usually rise, too.

Another important factor to consider with cholesterol levels is fiber intake. With the amount of fiber in fruit, vegetables, and salad, many people are able to significantly improve their cholesterol profile by reaching target fiber goals as well.

In general, it is much more hazardous for your health to eat too little protein than to eat protein from meat sources. Obviously, too much of a good thing is not a good thing, but most people with the **MD Factor** eat far more carbohydrates than protein, and that is one of the triggers for their condition.

Appendix B   Blood Work for the MD Factor

This is the comprehensive list of blood tests I order for each patient who wants to lose weight. They are the best way to give me all the details I need about how well their metabolism is functioning.

Complete blood count (CBC) This measures your red and white blood cell counts. It helps ensure that there are no immune system problems, such as an infection, or an iron deficiency problem, such as a low red blood cell count (anemia).

Complete metabolic panel (CMP) This chemistry profile measures your fasting blood glucose. It shows how your kidney and liver are functioning, as well as the levels of your electrolytes, including potassium, sodium, and calcium. Ideally, your fasting blood glucose should be around 75–85 mg/dL. Up to 99 is considered normal, but I consider fasting glucose levels in the mid-to-high 90s very suspicious for the **MD Factor**.

Thyroid-stimulating hormone (TSH) TSH is produced by the pituitary gland to tell your thyroid to make and release the hormones that regulate your metabolism. Assessing this level helps indicate whether or not your thyroid function is too high, too low, or normal.

T4, free This is a more specific thyroid test. T4 is an inactive hormone that is converted into the active thyroid hormone T3 when the body needs it.

T3, free Another specific thyroid test. If you have the **MD Factor**, you might have a problem converting inactive T4 into active T3, which would slow your metabolism down. T3 tells your cells to produce energy; low levels usually mean low energy, even if you are taking a synthetic T4 medication such as Synthroid.

Fasting serum insulin level Your fasting serum insulin level shows how well your body uses insulin to get glucose inside the cells that need it. If it's elevated, then you have the **MD Factor**. Many labs state that a value higher than 15 is abnormal, but many weight management experts, myself included, believe that a 6 or higher is abnormal.

Glycohemoglobin (HbA1c) This gives an indication of your average glucose level over a period of about ninety days, which is how long red blood cells live in your body. It measures how much sugar is attached to your red blood cells. When your red blood cells have higher than normal amounts of glucose saturating them, you have an elevated blood sugar and the **MD Factor**. I've found that your fasting blood sugar can be completely normal while the HbA1c can be higher than normal. This indicates that your blood sugar is higher than normal in the non-fasting state, which would be after you've eaten a meal. Different labs have different ranges of normal, but if you are out of range or at the upper limit of normal, you have the **MD Factor**. In our lab, we use the cut off of 5.5 percent as suspicious and 5.6 percent as definite for the **MD Factor**.

Lipid profile A lipid profile looks at your total cholesterol levels, both "good" HDL and "bad" LDL, and your triglycerides. This is a very powerful diagnostic tool for the **MD Factor**, as elevated triglycerides are an early sign that you have it. While many labs consider triglycerides to be normal if they are less than 150, I believe that a level over 100 is suspicious for the **MD Factor**. Low HDL is also a powerful sign for it, too.

25-OH vitamin D level This is the active form of vitamin D3 in your bloodstream. Vitamin D deficiency is found at a level below 20–30, depending on your lab. A more ideal level is between 36–42, and many people may need supplementation with active vitamin D3 in order to reach it.

Magnesium RBC This test measures the amount of magnesium inside your red blood cells, which is the most sensitive marker for a deficiency. I recommend this test over a serum (outside of the cell) magnesium level, as levels of magnesium inside cells can decline significantly before a deficiency can be picked up on a serum blood test.

Your physician must specify "red blood cell magnesium level" for the proper test to be done.

Serum vitamin B12 This measures the amount of vitamin B12 you have available in your bloodstream. Vitamin B12 is necessary for maintaining good energy levels and for your body's proper glucose regulation. It also plays a large role in proper nerve function and aids circulation.

Calculating Net Carbohydrates

Appendix C

To calculate net carbohydrates for a food, take the total carbohydrates and subtract fiber and sugar alcohols, if present, from this number. What you have left are the carbohydrates that actually raise your blood sugar. Be mindful of food labels until you are more familiar with net carbs, because not all carbohydrate foods contain fiber or sugar alcohols. Prunes have sugar alcohols, for instance, but peanuts do not. Food manufacturers will add fiber and sugar alcohols to their nutrition label so that consumers can tally net carbohydrates. Sugar alcohols, if present, will be listed in the nutrition panel as sugar alcohols or sugar alc.

This is a typical nutrition label for baby carrots:

To calculate net carbohydrates, take the total carbohydrates and subtract both fiber and sugar alcohols. Carrots do not contain sugar alcohols so just subtract the dietary fiber. Then record the net carbohydrates in your food log and add them up through the day.

Nutrition Facts

Serving size: 3 ounces
Servings in container: 1

Amount Per Serving

Total Fat 0 g

Saturated Fat 0 g

Trans Fat 0 g

Cholesterol 0 mg

Sodium 66 mg

Total Carbohydrate 7 g

Dietary Fiber 2 g

Sugars 4 g

Protein 1g

Ingredients: Carrots

Three ounces of baby carrots contain 5 grams of net carbohydrates.

	7 grams total carbohydrate
−	2 grams of dietary fiber
=	5 grams net carbs

Remember, most foods have at least a few carbohydrates in them. In a typical restaurant salad loaded with different items, these carbs quickly add up. For example, sliced tomatoes add about 2 grams of net carbs. Add the croutons or tortilla strips, the salad dressing, mandarin oranges or dried cranberries, and candied pecans, and you are already past 20 grams in a meal that appears to be very low in carbohydrates.

One other important point: some people with the **MD Factor** can tolerate more carbohydrates than others, eating more carbs per meal once in a while and still losing weight. Others need to be much stricter. It all depends on how high your **MD Factor** is and how quickly your system responds to the **MD Factor** Action Plan.

Genetic Influences on Your Weight

Appendix D

Much of the research about weight and metabolism looks at changes in our environment—how, as a country, we are consuming more calories and more sugars and are moving less in our daily lives.

An equally large body of research has been done to identify genes that predispose people to gaining weight and becoming too heavy. Many studies were done by researchers that showed how people with a certain gene variant would have faulty biochemical signaling telling them whether or not they were full after eating a meal. Those with that gene variant would eat more, as they don't respond to normal satiety signals.

To be honest, the more I studied the complexity of weight and the many different factors affecting our bodies' ability to regulate it, the more pessimistic I felt that people who struggle with weight could ever lose it and keep it off. I truly understood how my patients were struggling. They were highly motivated and following directions, but something still wasn't working. Now, of course, the **MD Factor** Action Plan works extremely well even if someone has had years of weight issues. But I'm still intrigued by the genetic factors that my patients have no control over.

In 2013, I became aware of a new type of genetic test called Pathway Fit, which provides a personal genetic report specific to diet, nutrition, and exercise. All you need to provide is a small sample of saliva from which DNA is extracted. From it, 140 different genes are evaluated that affect weight, eating behavior, the response of the body to exercise, and the metabolism of certain substances such as alcohol and caffeine. Other genes are evaluated that reveal a predisposition to having lower levels of certain vitamins, which we know influence both health *and* weight. This DNA analysis shows that a more personalized approach to nutrition and weight management is theoretically possible. I decided to submit my DNA for the test and see what it meant for me.

The Pathway Fit results are scored with a scientific strength rating, from one star to four stars, and relate to how strong the scientific studies were that prove the result conclusions. A four-star rating is given to gene information that has come from a study involving at least two thousand people and when at least one other study has replicated these findings. It means that this genetic information and its interpretation regarding nutrition and weight is quite strong. A one-star rating indicates the information found in specific genes is weaker, because it came from a smaller study and those results have not been replicated.

When my results arrived, my DNA spoke volumes about my weight management, nutritional tendencies, and best forms of exercise. The most striking piece of information was that my Obesity Index—which factors in the genes that influence whether or not I develop obesity—is high. In fact, there are five different risk ratings, which include low, below average, average, above average, and high, and I fall into the highest range. Nine different genes that have variants that predispose to obesity were tested, and the scientific strength supporting these genes was very strong.

I was partly surprised by this rating, but it also partly validated my interest in this field. I gravitated toward a practice emphasizing weight management due to my own personal interest, as I come from a family with weight problems. All of my immediate family members have struggled with weight, as did almost all of my grandparents. I remember reading in medical school that if both parents were obese, the child had an 80 percent likelihood of becoming obese. This fact really stuck with me.

As a teenager, I was determined not to become overweight, so I became more aware of my diet and started exercising regularly. There was plenty of good-natured teasing from my family as I did aerobics in our basement when I was in high school. At the University of Miami, I was in an accelerated program that allowed me to complete college and medical school in six years. It was intense, but I refused to quit my aerobics. After

I'd sat in a dark lecture hall for eight hours, a loud, bright aerobic dance class cleared my head enough to enable me to study for three to four more hours at night.

My regular routine of intense cardiovascular and weight training five to six times a week kept me slim, and as I learned more and more about the intricacies of nutrition and exercise, I have become even more fit. I knew that a lot of this was from my lifestyle choices, but I wondered if I—unlike my family members—had simply dodged a bullet and did not inherit the genes that predispose to obesity, because maintaining my weight has always been easy for me.

So the genetic test has answered a huge question for me. I did not just get lucky or dodge a genetic bullet. My lifestyle choices have kept my obesity genes from being expressed. I still have these genes, but I am not overweight thanks to my diet and exercise. DNA testing made me realize that paying attention to my exercise and diet is something I will always need to do. My health depends on it.

You Can Defeat Obesity Genes with Exercise

My DNA tests showed that exercise will enhance my ability to lose weight and increase my cells' sensitivity to insulin. This is great news, because a problem with impaired insulin sensitivity is what triggers the **MD Factor**. I didn't know it then, but when I started doing aerobics in high school, my lifestyle change counteracted my genetic predisposition to being overweight. If I hadn't exercised and stuck to a careful diet, I likely wouldn't have stayed so slim. I know many people who have been very restrictive with their diet but didn't exercise, and they struggle with their weight.

Genetics Affect Your Taste Buds

DNA testing also looks at how you respond to certain foods and whether or not you are a "bitter taster" or a "nontaster." Tasters have a genetic variant that make certain foods taste more bitter, and the best example are vegetables such as broccoli. Some children find vegetables to be much more bitter than other children do—and they aren't faking. It's a recipe for family stress.

I tested two of my children and found that one was a taster and one wasn't—which I already knew after feeding them for years. This information is helpful because strong bitter tasters need to seek out vegetables they do like, and they might need to take some supplements to ensure they get all the vitamins they may miss from the bitter foods they avoid.

The Pathway Fit profile also looks for genetic predispositions toward certain eating behaviors. There are genes associated with snacking, hunger, satiety, food desire, sweet tooth, and eating disinhibition. Someone with genes that show a predisposition for eating disinhibition should not buy a half gallon of ice cream and convince themselves they won't eat too much or all of it. They'd do much better by only getting a single portion of ice cream at a shop. A person with this issue may also do better with the 100-calorie packs for treats rather than a larger box. I do have the gene for eating disinhibition, but it's never been an issue for me. Of course, my career involves treating and preventing weight problems, so I suspect that I had a tendency toward this behavior when younger and extinguished it with conscious effort!

Vitamins and Genetics

I was very excited to see what the genetic information revealed about vitamin status. The test looked at a predisposition to having lower blood levels of several vitamins, specifically vitamin B6, vitamin B12, folic acid, vitamin A, vitamin D, and vitamin E. In my medical practice I test specific nutrients because I find that when people have lower levels of them, it is harder to lose weight. Specifically, low vitamin D and B12 are associated with the **MD Factor**, as you know. Monitoring these vitamin levels and supplementing with appropriate vitamins is a helpful adjunctive treatment for my patients who struggle with weight.

I've monitored my own vitamin levels for several years and know that I need to take fairly high doses of vitamin D to move into the normal and optimal range. I also found that my levels of the B vitamins were low. My genetic tests showed that my genetic variants are associated with lower levels of vitamin D, vitamin B6, folate, and vitamin E. This was very helpful for me, as I have wondered why my body needed so much more of certain nutrients. It also explains why you can be nutrient deficient even when you eat a healthful, balanced diet. Our bodies genetically differ in our ability to absorb, metabolize, and transport these nutrients into our cells, and some of us will always need supplements, no matter how well we eat.

The Best Diet for Your Genetics

My DNA tests also recommended the best type of diet for my body, either low-carb, low-fat, balanced, or Mediterranean. This would help all dieters who don't know what to eat, because there are so many contradictory diet plans out there.

Genetic testing looked at how the body responds to monounsaturated fats, like olive oil, or polyunsaturated fats, like vegetable oils. Someone who benefits from monounsaturated fats would do better on a Mediterranean diet. They also looked at the genetic variants that are associated with elevated LDL or "bad" cholesterol. Someone with a genetic likelihood toward high LDL would probably do better on a low-fat diet that would lower high LDL levels. Genetic variants associated with decreased HDL or "good" cholesterol, elevated triglycerides, and elevated blood sugar were also tested. An increased probability toward these three factors indicates a predisposition toward the **MD Factor**, so a low-carb diet would be best.

While this information is helpful, it's important to remember that genetic predisposition to certain blood chemistry markers such as cholesterol is not necessarily what might be going on in your body *now*. For example, I may have a patient with a genetic predisposition to do well on a balanced diet—but if she is having a very stressful time at work, stopped smoking, and hasn't been able to exercise, she may have gained thirty pounds, particularly in her belly. This, as you know, can trigger the **MD Factor**. She may also have higher triglycerides and low HDL even though the genetic analysis says otherwise. This patient will do best by initially following the **MD Factor** Action Plan to lose her visceral fat and lessen her **MD Factor**. Once she's at her ideal weight, a balanced diet would work very well.

Bear in mind, too, that while DNA testing is a helpful addition for my patients' evaluations, it's still not intended to be a replacement for a comprehensive weight management program, either with a physician or with this book. But it does help my patients feel a lot better about their weight struggles, particularly once they realize that they're overweight not simply because they ate too much or were lazy, as they might have been told by well-meaning or ill-informed friends, loved ones, and medical professionals. Body weight and weight regulation are highly complex and influenced by many different genes. You may have been born with factors out of your control, but the **MD Factor** Action Plan will put that control back in your capable hands.

Metformin

Sometimes my patients follow the **MD Factor** Action Plan, take their supplements, and exercise regularly, but their **MD Factor** is stubborn. It just doesn't want to let go.

Metformin is a well-researched, commonly used medication to treat people with diabetes. It's not a stimulant, but it often suppresses your appetite. It can help regulate your blood sugar throughout the day, which can help reduce cravings. And it is very effective at reversing the **MD Factor**, as well as proactively preventing diabetes from forming. Since metformin doesn't increase the amount of insulin you produce, it's less likely to cause low blood sugar, or hypoglycemia, as many other medications for diabetes can do. In fact, it's one of the few diabetes medications that doesn't cause weight gain—it actually helps most people *lose* weight.

Metformin works in three ways:

- It limits the amount of sugar produced by your liver. As you know, when you have the **MD Factor**, the sugar in your blood can't get into the cells where it's needed. Your body thinks it's starving and sends signals to your liver to produce more sugar. With metformin, however, those signals to your liver are blocked.

- It limits the amount of sugar your body absorbs whenever you eat.

- It helps your body respond better to its own insulin. As a result, your blood sugar levels will go down. The abnormal chemistry of the **MD Factor** starts to reverse. You won't feel so hungry all the time, and you won't be craving carbohydrates. Plus, you'll finally be able to lose weight.

That's what happened to Jennifer. "When Dr. Cederquist checked my blood sugar, it was elevated at 112, which is in the prediabetic range," she explains. "And my HbA1c was 6.0 percent, while normal is below

5.5 percent. My insulin level should have been 6 or below, but it was elevated at 24.

"I started the **MD Factor** Action Plan and finally was able to make some progress—I lost fourteen pounds in eight weeks and felt a lot better. Dr. Cederquist rechecked my lab tests then and was happy to see that my blood sugar was better at 102, but not normal yet. My insulin level actually went up to 29. Dr. Cederquist explained that despite my sticking to the Action Plan and my weight loss—which the body composition scale showed was all from fat—my **MD Factor** blood tests were still very abnormal. And Dr. Cederquist told me that with my family history (my mother is 57 and has been diabetic for a few years) and my ethnic background (my family is from Cuba), I am at higher risk for the **MD Factor** and have probably had it since high school.

"She recommended I start metformin, which has really helped. My weight is coming off faster and I especially notice that my waistline is getting smaller. I am also less hungry, with fewer cravings for sugars and starches. These cravings were already better with following the **MD Factor** Action Plan, and now I don't have any at all.

"As I'm planning to have another child in a few years, I checked with my ob/gyn, who agreed with Dr. Cederquist's care plan and advised me to continue the metformin. After only eight more weeks on the meal plan and metformin, I was able to lose 35 pounds."

Discuss the possibility of taking metformin with your physician. If you do take it, it can lower your vitamin B12 levels, so I recommend that you take 250–500 mcg of B12 as a supplement each day. Your doctor will best be able to advise you.

Appendix F

Nutrition Information Quick Reference Guide

Below is a list of the vegetables that are acceptable on your diet. Choose raw or frozen (thawed) with no sugar added. For serving sizes, remember that the serving of a cooked vegetable is half of the raw serving (1 cup raw = ½ cup cooked). The nutritional information below is calculated using the raw serving size unless otherwise noted.

	Serving Size	Protein (g)	Net Carbohydrates (g)	Fat (g)	Fiber (g)
Vegetables—Best Source of Carbohydrates					
Artichoke hearts	½ cup	3	4.5	0	4.5
Arugula, raw	2 cups	1	0.5	0	0.5
Asparagus	1 cup	2	0.5	0	1
Beans, green and wax	1 cup	2	4	0	4
Beets, cooked	½ cup	1.5	6.5	0	2
Broccoli	1 cup	2.5	2	0	2.5
Brussels sprouts	1 cup	3	5	0	3.5
Cabbage	1 cup	1.5	3	0	2
Carrots	½ cup	0.5	4	0	2
Cauliflower	1 cup	2	2.5	0	2.5
Celery	1 cup	1	2.5	0	2
Cucumber	1 cup	0.5	2	0	1
Eggplant	1 cup	1	3	0	2
Greens, collard, mustard, turnip	1 cup	1.5	1	0	4
Leeks	½ cup	0.5	5.5	0	1
Mushrooms, raw	1 cup	3	1.5	1.5	0.5
Okra	½ cup	2	2.5	0	5

	Serving Size	Protein (g)	Net Carbohydrates (g)	Fat (g)	Fiber (g)
Onion	½ cup	1	4.5	0	1.5
Pepper, red or green, raw	½ cup	0.5	3	0	1
Radish, raw	10	Trace	1	0	0.5
Romaine lettuce	2 cups	2	1	0	2
Shallots	½ cup	1	6	0	0
Snow peas	½ cup	2	3	0	2
Spinach, cooked	1 cup	2.5	1	0	2
Spinach, raw	2 cups	3	1	0	3
Sauerkraut	1 cup	2	4	0	5.5
Spaghetti squash, cooked	½ cup	0.5	4	0	1
Sprouts, alfalfa	1 cup	1.5	0.5	0	1
Sprouts, mung bean	1 cup	2	2.5	0	0.5
Summer squash, raw	1 cup	1	3	0	2.5
Swiss chard, boiled	½ cup	1.5	2	0	2
Tomato	1 small	1	4	0	1.5
Zucchini	1 cup	1	1.5	0	1

Legumes: Beans, Peas, and Starchy Squash

	Serving Size	Protein (g)	Net Carbohydrates (g)	Fat (g)	Fiber (g)
Black beans, cooked	½ cup	7.5	12.5	0.5	7.5
Chickpeas, cooked	½ cup	6	22	1.5	5
Kidney beans, cooked	½ cup	6.5	14.5	0.5	4.5
Lentils, cooked	½ cup	9	12	0.5	8
Lima beans, cooked	½ cup	6	12	Trace	6
Pinto beans, cooked	½ cup	6	12	1	6.5
Split peas, cooked	½ cup	8	12.5	0.5	8
Pigeon peas, cooked	½ cup	5.5	9.5	Trace	6.5
Black-eyed peas (cowpeas), cooked	½ cup	7	14	0.5	4
Acorn squash	½ cup	1	10.5	0	4.5
Butternut squash	½ cup	1.5	12	0	1

*The **MD Factor** Diet*

	Serving Size	Protein (g)	Net Carbohydrates (g)	Fat (g)	Fiber (g)
Cereals and Breads					
High fiber cereals	½ – ¾ cup	2–4	8–18	1–1.5	10–14
Protein-supplemented cereal	½ – ¾ cup	10	9	3	5
100% whole-wheat bread	1 slice	3–4	8–10	1	2
Whole-wheat English muffin	½ muffin	3	11	0.5	2
Low-carb wrap	1 wrap	9	8	2.5	9
Low-carb pita	1 pita	6	4	2	4
Fruits					
Choose fresh, frozen, or canned (without sugar or heavy syrup)					
Apples	1 (2.5 in. diameter)	0	17	0.5	4
Applesauce, unsweetened	½ cup	0	14	0	2
Apricots, dried	4 halves	0.5	7	0	1
Apricots, fresh	2 medium	1	6.5	0	1.5
Banana	½ medium	0.5	12.5	0.5	1.5
Blackberries	⅔ cup	1	7.5	0.5	5
Blueberries	⅔ cup	1	11	0.5	2.5
Boysenberries	⅔ cup	1	7	0	3.5
Cantaloupe	¼ (6 in. diameter)	1	10.5	0	1
Cherries	10	1	10.5	0.5	1.5
Clementines	1 med/3 oz.	0	15	0	1
Dates	2	0	11	0	1
Grapefruit	½ small	0.5	8	0	1.5
Grapes	15	0.5	12.5	0.5	1
Honeydew, cubed	½ cup	0.5	7.5	0	0.5
Kiwi	1 medium	1	8	0	2.5
Mandarin oranges	½ cup	1	11	0	1

	Serving Size	Protein (g)	Net Carbohydrates (g)	Fat (g)	Fiber (g)
Mango, cubed	½ cup	0.5	12.5	0	1.5
Nectarine	1 medium	1	14	0.5	2
Orange	1 small	1	12.5	0	3
Papaya, cubed	½ cup	0.5	6	0	1
Peach	1 medium	0.5	9	0	2
Pear, Bartlett	½ small	0	10.5	0	2
Persimmon	1	0	8	0	0
Pineapple, cubed	½ cup	0	9	0	1
Plum	1 medium	0.5	7.5	0	1
Raspberries	⅔ cup	1	4	0.5	5.5
Strawberries	1 cup	1	7	0.5	3
Tangerine	1 medium	0.5	7.5	0	2
Watermelon, cubed	1 cup	1	11	0	1

Whole Grains and Starchy Vegetables

	Serving Size	Protein (g)	Net Carbohydrates (g)	Fat (g)	Fiber (g)
Whole-wheat macaroni, cooked	½ cup	4	16.5	0.5	2
Whole-wheat spaghetti, cooked	½ cup	4	15.5	0.5	3
Couscous, cooked	½ cup	3.5	20	Trace	1.5
Brown rice, cooked	½ cup	2	21.5	0.5	1.5
Wild rice, cooked	½ cup	3	17	Trace	0.75

*The **MD Factor** Diet*

	Serving Size	Protein (g)	Net Carbohydrates (g)	Fat (g)	Fiber (g)
Baked potato with skin	3 oz	1.5	20.5	0	1.5
Baked sweet potato with skin	3 oz	1.5	18.5	0	2.5
Mashed potatoes	½ cup	2	15.5	4	2
Oat bran bagel	½ bagel	4	18	1	1
Whole-wheat pita, 6-in. diameter	½ pita	3	15	1	2.5
Whole-wheat tortilla	1 tortilla	4	24	2.5	2
Whole-wheat roll	1 small	2.5	12.5	1	2
Whole-wheat bread	1 slice	4	10	1	2
Corn	½ cup	2	13.5	1	1.5
Quinoa	¼ cup	5.5	27	2.5	2.5
Oatmeal	¼ cup	3	11.5	1.3	2

Appendix G MD Factor Food Log

	Protein (g)	Net Carbs (g)	Fat (g)
Breakfast			
Protein			
Fruit or grain (T&S Days only)			
Beverage			
Snack			
Lunch			
Protein			
Non-starchy vegetable(s)			
Fruit or grain (T&S Days only)			
Beverage			
Snack			
Dinner			
Protein			
Non-starchy vegetable(s)			
Fruit or grain (S Days only)			
Beverage			
Snack			
DAILY TOTAL			

Additional Resources

There are many additional resources that I can offer you to help you live a more healthy life. Here are a few for you to add to your routine now.

Try bistroMD If you want to follow the **MD Factor** but need help in the kitchen, try bistroMD. I created bistroMD, a home diet delivery program, to provide access nationwide to delicious, chef-prepared entrees that are made to my unique specifications for weight loss and to treat Metabolism Dysfunction.

BistroMD is a labor of love, as the meals are created with high-quality ingredients without nitrates, phosphates, other chemicals or additives, or even the ridiculously and dangerously high sodium levels frequently found in frozen or other convenience meals. My philosophy has been that if I won't eat it or feel good about feeding it to my children or my patients, there is no way it will be allowed onto the bistroMD menu! For more information, go to www.bistroMD.com.

Keep in Contact Go online to my website, www.DrCederquist.com and sign up for my newsletter to receive free health information, recipes, and healthy living resources delivered to your inbox.

Go Social! Follow me on Facebook, Twitter, and Google+.

Learn More To learn more, check out the health articles on my website. These excellent resources are just a click away!

How bistroMD is Different

Readers of *The **MD Factor** Diet* may notice that the bistroMD diet delivery program differs slightly from the **MD Factor** Action Plan outlined in this book. The Action Plan has been designed to provide the average person with the greatest chance of achieving life-transforming wellness through the reversal of metabolism dysfunction. BistroMD members, as well as patients in my practice, will notice slight departures from the Action Plan in this book due to the ability in both cases for individualized customization of programs. Rest assured, in both the **MD Factor** Action Plan, as well as the bistroMD diet delivery plan, users will receive the full range of benefits that result when they retrain their dysfunctional metabolism.

Appendix I   Animal Protein and Vegetarian Diets

Being overweight, especially if one is 30 percent above their ideal weight, is a strong risk factor for the increased development of many types of cancer. Being diabetic, which is an advanced form of the **MD Factor**, also increases the risk of many types of cancer.

Cancer is a significant health concern. Several popular books have communicated the increased risk of cancer in populations with a higher intake of animal-based protein. To lose weight and also have an increase in overall health and wellness, I find it is most critical to first correct the metabolic dysfunction that makes weight gain so easy and weight loss so challenging. This involves the intake of a lower calorie diet that contains adequate lean protein and controlled carbohydrate and fat intake.

The control of carbohydrate intake is crucial to lower insulin levels. Recall that high insulin levels promote fat storage. Also, high insulin levels can cause reactive hypoglycemia, which induces physical hunger and sweet cravings that sabotage willpower and contribute to the ongoing cycle of weight gain. Animal protein contains a higher amount of protein coupled with lower carbohydrate content. This is why I recommend animal-based protein in the weight loss process. Although you can obtain protein from vegetarian meals such as beans and rice, the carbohydrate content of the meal will be three to five times the protein content. Many people with the **MD Factor** cannot reverse their condition with this higher carbohydrate intake.

Metabolic dysfunction is both treatable and reversible with an adequate lean protein and controlled carbohydrate diet. As you correct metabolic dysfunction, you can replace animal-based proteins with more vegetarian choices because your tolerance for carbohydrates increases. I support correcting the metabolic abnormalities we know are associated with increased cancer risk and then transitioning this successful meal plan to one that incorporates more vegetarian protein and less animal protein for long-term weight maintenance and optimal health.

References

Albarracin et al. Chromium picolinate and biotin combination improves glucose metabolism in treated, uncontrolled overweight to obese patients with type 2 diabetes. *Diabetes Metab Res Rev.* 2008; 24: 41–51.

Anderson, Harvey, Shannon Moore. Dietary proteins in the regulation of food intake and body weight in human. *J. Nutr.* 2004; 134(4): 974S–979S.

Carr, Molly C. The emergence of the metabolic syndrome with menopause. *J Clin Endocrinol Metab.* 2003; 88: 2404–2411.

Conn, Jerome W., H. S. Seltzer. Spontaneous hypoglycemia. *Am J Med.* 1955; 19(3): 460–478.

Crawford, Peter. Effectiveness of cinnamon for lowering hemoglobin AIC in patients with type 2 diabetes: a randomized, controlled trial. *J Am Board Fam Med.* 2009; 22: 507–512.

Davies, et al. Hormones, weight change and menopause. *Int J Obes Relat Metab Disord.* 2001 June; 25(6): 874–879.

Donato et al. Association between menopause status and central adiposity measured at different cutoffs of weight circumference and waist-to-hip ratio. *Menopause* 2006; 13: 280–285.

Ervin et al. Prevalence of metabolic syndrome among adults 20 years of age and over, by sex, age, race and ethnicity, and body mass index: United States, 2003–2006. *Natl Health Stat Report.* 2009 May; (13): 1–7.

Fink R. et al. Mechanisms of Insulin Resistance in Aging. *J Clin Invest.* June 1983; 71(6): 1523–35.

Halton, Thomas et al. The effects of high protein diets on thermogenesis, satiety and weight loss: A critical review. *J Am Coll Nutr.* 2004; 23(5): 373–285.

Havel, Peter, PhD. Dietary fructose: implications for dysregulation of energy homeostasis and lipid/carbohydrate metabolism. *Nutr Rev.* 2005 May; 63(5): 113–57.

Heaney, Robert P., Donald Layman. Amount and type of protein influences bone health. *Am J Clin Nutr.* 2008; 87(5): 1567S– 1570S.

Holick, M. et al., Prevalence of vitamin D inadequacy among postmenopausal north american women receiving osteoporosis therapy. *J Clin Endocrinol Metab.* 2005; 90(6): 3215–3224.

Hudspeth WJ, et al. Neurobiology of the hypoglycemia syndrome. *J Holistic Med* 1981; 3(1): 60–71

Kamenova, Petya. Improvement of insulin sensitivity in patients with type 2 diabetes mellitus after oral administration of alpha-lipoic acid. *Hormones (Athens).* 2006 Oct–Dec; 5(4): 251–258.

Kelly, Gregory S N.D. Clinical applications of N-acetylcysteine. *Alt Med Rev* 1998; 3(2): 114–127.

Kidd, Parris. Bioavailability and activity of phytosome complexes and botanical polyphenols: the silymarin, curcumin, green tea, and grape seed extracts. *Altern Med Rev.* 2009; 14(3): 226–246.

Knekt, P. et al., Serum vitamin D and subsequent occurrence of type 2 diabetes. *Epidemiology.* 2008; 19(5): 666–671.

Koh et al. Effects of alpha-lipoic acid on body weight in obese subjects. *Am J Med.* 2011; 124(1): 85e1–85e8.

Layman, Donald K. Protein quantity and quality at levels above the RDA improves adult weight loss. *J Am Coll Nutr.* 2004; 23(6): 631–636.

Layman, Donald K. et al. Protein in optimal health: heart disease and type 2 diabetes. *Am J Clin Nutr.* 2008; 87(5): 87.

Layman, Donald K., Jamie Baum. Dietary protein impact on glycemic control during weight loss. *J. Nutr.* 2004; 134(4): 968S–973S.

Lemay et al. Hyperinsulinemia in non-obese women reporting a moderate weight gain at the beginning or menopause: a useful early measure of susceptibility to insulin resistance. *Menopause.* 2010 March; 17: 321–325.

Li CI, Malone KE, Porter PL, Weiss NS, Tang MT, Daling JR. The relationship between alcohol use and risk of breast cancer by histology and hormone receptor status among women 65–79 years of age. *Cancer Epidemiol Biomarkers Prev.* 2003; 12: 1061–1066.

Li. et. al., Effects of multivitamin and mineral supplementation on adiposity, energy expenditure and lipid profiles in obese Chinese women. *Int J Obes* (Lond). 2010; 24: 1070–1077.

Liu, E. et al., Plasma 25-hydroxyvitamin D is associated with markers of the insulin resistant phenotype in nondiabetic adults, *J Nutr.* 2009; 139(2): 329–334.

Lovejoy, Jennifer. The menopause and obesity. *Primary Care Clin Office Pract.* 2003; 20: 317–325.

Millea, PJ., N-acetylecystiene: Multiple clinical applications. *Am Fam Physician.* 2009 Aug 1; 80(3): 265–269.

Mozaffarian D, Katan MB, Ascherio A, Stampfer MJ, Willett WC. Trans fatty acids and cardiovascular disease. *N Engl J Med.* 2006; 354:1; 601–1613.

Musatov S, W. Chen, D. Clegg, et al. Silencing of estrogen receptor alpha in the ventromedial nucleus of hypothalamus leads to metabolic syndrome. *Proc Natl Acad Sci USA*. 2007; 104(7); 2501–2506.

Nagao T, Meguro S, Hase T, et al. A catechins-rich beverage improves obesity and blood glucose control in patients with Type 2 diabetes. *Obesity* (Silver Spring). 2009; 17: 310–317.

Nedungadi T, D. Clegg. Sexual dimoprhism in body fat distribution and risk for cardiovascular diseases. *J Cardiovasc Transl Res*. 2009; 2: 321–327.

Noakes, Manny et al. Effect of an energy-restricted, high protein, low fat diet relative to a conventional high-carbohydrate, low–fat diet on weight loss, body composition, nutritional status and markers of cardiovascular health in obese women. *Am J Clin Nutr*. 2005; 81: 1298–306.

Optimal serum 25-hydroxyvitamin D levels for multiple health outcomes. *Adv Exp Med Biol.*; 2008; 624: 55–71.

Park et al. The metabolic syndrome: prevalence and associated risk factor findings in the US population from the third national health and nutrition examination survey, 1988–1994. *Arch Intern Med*. 2003; 163: 427–436.

Pasquali et al. Body weight, fat distribution and the menopausal status in women. The VMH Collaborative Group. *Int J Obes Relat Metab Disord*. 1994; 18: 614–621.

Pepino, M.Y. et al. Sucralose affects glycemic and hormonal responses to an oral glucose load. *Diabetes Care*. 2013; 36(9): 2530–35.

Qin B, M. Nagasaki, M. Ren, G. Bajotto, Y. Oshida, Y. Sato. Cinnamon extract prevents the insulin resistance induced by a high-fructose diet. *Horm Metab Res*. 2004 Feb; 36(2): 119–25.

Roepke, Troy A. Oestrogen modulates hypothalamic control of energy homeostasis through multiple mechanisms. *J Neuroendocrinol*. 2009 February; 21(2): 141–150.

Soenen S et al. Normal protein intake is required for body weight loss and weight maintenance, and elevated protein intake for additional preservation of resting energy expenditure and fat free mass. *J Nutr*. 2013; 143(5): 591–596.

Toth et al. Effect of menopausal status on body composition and abdominal fat distribution. *Int J Obes Relat Metab Disord*. 2000; 24: 226–231.

Van Proeyen K, K. Szlufcik et al. Training in the fasted state improves glucose tolerance during fat-rich diet. *J Physiol*. 2010 Nov 1; 588(Pt21): 4289–302.

Volek, JS et al. Carbohydrate restriction has a more favorable impact on the metabolic syndrome than a low fat diet. *Lipids*. 2009; 44(4): 297–309

Walker Lasker, Denise et al. Moderate carbohydrate, moderate protein weight loss diet reduces cardiovascular disease risk compared to high carbohydrate, low protein diet in obese adults: A randomized clinical trial. *Nutr Metab* (Lond). 2008; 30(5).

Wang, et al. Total and regional body-composition changes in early postmenopausal women: age-related or menopause-related? *Am J Clin Nutrition* 1994; 60: 843–848.

Welsh, S. A. Calorie sweetener consumption and dyslipidemia among US adults. *JAMA*. 2010; 303(15): 1490–1497.

Wing RR, et al. Weight gain at the time of menopause. *Arch Intern Med* 1991; 151: 97–102.

Zhang, Cuilin et al. Abdominal obesity and the risk if all- cause cardiovascular and cancer mortality. sixteen years of follow-up in US women. *Circulation*. 2009; 1117: 1658–1667

Utian, WH et al. Estrogen and progestogen use in postmenopausal women: July 2008 position statement of The North American Menopause Society. *Menopause*. 2008; 15(4): 584–602.

Tuomilehto, J et al. Prevention of type 2 diabetes mellitus by changes in lifestyle among subjects with impaired glucose tolerance. *N Engl J Med*. 2001 May 3; 344(18): 1343–50.